W9-AXN-475

THE YOGA OF HERBS

AN AYURVEDIC GUIDE TO HERBAL MEDICINE

Second Revised & Enlarged Edition

by DR. DAVID FRAWLEY and
DR. VASANT LAD

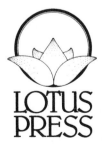

LOTUS
PRESS

Twin Lakes, Wisconsin

DISCLAIMER

This book is a reference work not intended to treat, diagnose or prescribe. The information contained herein is in no way to be considered as a substitute for consultation with a duly licensed health-care professional.

COPYRIGHT © 1986, 2001 BY DR. FRAWLEY & DR. VASANT LAD

ALL RIGHTS RESERVED. No part of this book may be reproduced in any form or by any electronic or mechanical means including information storage and retrieval systems without permission in writing from the publisher, except by a reviewer who may quote brief passages in a review.

PASSAGES TRANSLATED FROM THE SANSKRIT BY DAVID FRAWLEY

SECOND REVISED & ENLARGED EDITION, 2001
REPRINTED 2008

Printed in the United States of America

Library of Congress Cataloging-in-Publication Data

Lad, Vasant, 1943
   The Yoga of Herbs.

   Includes bibliographies and index.
   1. Herbs–Therapeutic use. 2. Medicine
   Ayurvedic. I. Frawley, David. II. Title.
   [DNLM: 1. Herbs 2. Medicine, Ayurvedic.
   3. Medicine Herbal. WB 925L153y]
RM666.H33L33 1986   615'.321'0954   86-81365
ISBN 978-0-9415-2424-7 (pbk.)

Published in 2001 by Lotus Press / P.O. Box 325 / Twin Lakes, WI 53181 www.lotuspress.com

DEDICATION

This book is dedicated to Lenny Blank, as it was through his effort, direction, foresight and perseverance that it was both begun and completed, as part of his continuing endeavor to help spread Ayurveda to the West.

CONTENTS

TABLE, CHART AND DIAGRAMS

ACKNOWLEDGMENTS

Santosh Krinsky   for his consistent support, without which this book could not have been produced.

Lavon Alt   typist, who produced the index. She is an Herbalist who made an invaluable contribution by helping to organize this book.

Angela Werneke   artist, who is responsible for all the art contained in this book, including the cover, diagrams and illustrations. Angela's work has greatly enhanced the quality of this book.

Mina Yamashita   responsible for the layout and production of the book, as well as the cover design. We appreciate her technical skill and creative involvement, which exceeded our expectations.

Ed Tarabilda   for his input in the generation of ideas that served as a background for this book.

Gerald Hausman   Editor

Laura Ware   Copy Editor

Casa Sin Nombre   Typesetter

PREFACE

The term "yoga" has many traditional meanings. In Ayurveda, the medical science of India, yoga refers to the "right usage" and "right combination" of herbs. A special combination of substances designed to bring about a specific effect upon the body or mind is thus called a "yoga ."

This coordinated or integrated usage of herbs was based upon the ancient Ayurvedic science of herbal energetics. In this is a system for determining the qualities and powers of herbs according to the laws of nature, so that herbs can be used objectively and specifically according to individual conditions. A yogic usage of herbs implies such an harmonic application of the potencies of herbs.

In this book, for the first time, this Ayurvedic herbal science is applied to western herbs, as well as to a few major oriental herbs, both Indian and Chinese. It is the purpose of this book not to present Ayurveda in the distance, as something foreign or ancient, but to make it a practically applied system of herbalism.

We live in a very special, yet very dangerous time, wherein a new global culture is painfully struggling to be born. It is the challenge of our times to integrate human culture and knowledge. It is essential that this process occurs on the level of the healing sciences also. Healing is always a matter of unification. If our healing knowledge cannot be integrated, how can we as human beings find unity among ourselves?

Ayurveda is an eternal system that has already integrated eight limbs of healing within itself, from herbs to surgery to psychology. As such it offers such a point of unification. Its very basis is the spiritual knowledge of the ancient seers of India and the cosmic consciousness in which they lived.

This book is not just a presentation of traditional Ayurvedic knowledge. It attempts to show living Ayurveda, its creative and practical application to changing conditions. It is meant as a bridge between east and west. In this regard, it has been a collaboration of an easterner with profound knowledge of the west and a westerner with profound knowledge of the east. It is our deepest wish that it transmits this spirit of integration and collaboration.

In the application of Ayurveda to the west, most traditional Ayurvedic medicines cannot be practically used. They may consist of special tropical herbs that are largely inaccessible here, or they may contain special mineral substances that can only be used after long and difficult preparations. Hence this book has arisen as a vehicle to make the healing knowledge of Ayurveda applicable to substances that are accessible and possess few potential side-effects.

At the same time, we have also attempted to preserve the integrality of the Ayurvedic healing system. For this we have included special effects of herbs upon the mind, and the deeper psychological and spiritual aspects of healing. Herbalism is part of this broader context of healing and without addressing these deeper issues of human life, no healing process can really be effective.

Sanskrit terms have been kept to a minimum and have been provided with easily understandable translations. For further elucidation of some of the medical concepts in this book, the reader is referred to *Ayurveda, the Science of Self-Healing,* which is a companion volume to it.

The classification of western herbs into eastern energetics is not something that can be done once and for all. Even in Ayurveda differences of classification of herbs sometimes exist between different writers. So we welcome any comments or criticism in this regard and invite all who wish to join us in this work to contact us.

We would like to express our most heartfelt gratitude to the many people, friends and students, who have served as a help and an inspiration to this book, as well as to the many others who are working in a similar direction. May their labors be fruitful.

> Dr. David Frawley
> Dr. Vasant Lad
> May, 1986
> Santa Fe, New Mexico

FOREWORD

As an herbalist with over 18 years of experience using Western, Chinese and Ayurvedic herbs, I long ago came to the conclusion that without taking into account the overall energetics of herbs and foods in relation to individual constitutional differences, we are bound for tremendous inconsistency and failure. Such an approach keeps us from drawing broad useful conclusions necessary for the prevention and cure of disease. In this, biochemistry alone is simply not enough.

There is much that can be shared between ancient healing systems of Eastern and Western science. Some, imbued with the Western scientific perspective, believe that ours is the most advanced and therefore the only true way. We fail to recognize that there are already, fully developed and theoretically articulated medical systems in India and China which have proven themselves effective for more than 3000 years. Ours, however, has only been developed over the past several hundred years.

Ayurvedic medicine is certainly one of the oldest systems with a consistent theoretical basis and practical clinical application. Into its ancient well of profound healing wisdom, some of the greatest doctors and sages have poured their finest insights and discoveries. Yet, to fully appreciate the nectar of this Eastern healing wisdom, Westerners need to overcome their literal and linear process of thought to enter into a non-linear reasoning approach. Therefore, a perspective grounded in an intuitive vision of the whole rather than the microscopic view of contemporary science is necessary.

The strength of Ayurveda lies in its broad, all-encompassing view of the dynamic interrelationship between organic physiological processes, external factors including climate, life work and diet along with internal emotional stages. In contrast, Western science takes a more particular view based upon specific molecular structure and chemistry. It is paradoxical that both could be describing the same condition in such different ways and with such diametrically opposed viewpoints.

Today, many people are drawn to Oriental healing systems and herbology because these approaches offer the promise of a healing system that is at once powerfully effective and gentle with the least danger of side effects. They rightly feel that disease occurs not as an arbitrary phenomenon but for definite reasons which if correctly understood could help to cure and more importantly, prevent recurrence.

Ayurveda, with its *Tridosha* or three humours system, is able to provide a complete understanding of the cause of health in terms of a metabolic balance. Disease is simply understood as an imbalance between the nerve energy (*vata*), catabolic fire energy (*pitta*) and anabolic nutritive energy (*kapha*). All foods and experiences have an effect on the overall balance of these respective humours. This is proven by the fact that through adjusting the balance of diet only, many health problems are alleviated (this is unfortunately still not considered a fact by the majority of Western-trained medical doctors).

Herbs are used as "special foods", serving to eliminate excesses and strengthen deficiencies. While they may possess a powerful nutritive impact on a weakened body, their primary action is to stimulate particular organic functions. This is the more illusive energetic aspect of herbs and indeed of all medicines, drugs and foods that need to be understood. Besides the specific function of a medicine or food, there is a more general effect in that for some who are predisposed, it can, broadly speaking, either raise or lower overall metabolism and stimulate or sedate nerve, nutritive or fire energies which comprise the *Tridosha* humoural system.

The fundamental error of western medicine is to treat the disease rather than the patient. If drugs were prescribed sensitively according to the individual nature of each person, as herbs are in Oriental healing systems, many of the side effects that result could be avoided. The value of using herbs and foods lies particularly in their relative non-specific action or their "mildness." If one misuses an herb, the results are relatively minor and are generally completed in the short span within a day or so that it takes for the body to eliminate the residues of the herb from the system. It is more difficult with synthetic drugs or extracted concentrates. The liver may be unable to fully eliminate a drug from the tissues and cells of the body because it has not figured out how to neutralize it either for assimilation or elimination. Unable to fully process the substance, it is stored in the liver and tissues or circulates in the body, creating a toxic burden that impairs necessary organic physiological processes.

Before one can fully realize the healing benefits of Ayurveda or Chinese medicine, both of which are "energetic" systems of healing, all foods and herbs must be classified and understood in terms of their broader energetic effects on overall metabolic processes. I believe that Dr. David Frawley's and Dr. Vasant Lad's book successfully, for the first time, offers such a classification of herbs, including Western herbs and herbs common to both East and West. It is of coincidence that this manuscript should find its way into my hands just at the time that I have nearly completed my own research into classifying Western herbs into the traditional Chinese energetic system. It is also fascinating to see how, in many instances, their method of classification and my own demonstrate the same basic energetic understanding.

Dr. David Frawley and Dr. Lad have made a truly powerful and unique contribution to alternative, natural health care by their creation of this important book. It may take a while for the majority of non-Ayurvedically oriented people to see the practical benefits of this original work. However, it is simply the difference between a hit and miss approach, and the development of a consistent and valid herbal healing system.

This book for the first time will serve not only to make Ayurvedic medicine of greater practical value to Westerners, but in fact, ultimately advance the whole system of Western herbalism forward into greater effectiveness. I think anyone interested in herbs should closely study this book whether their interests lie in Western herbology, traditional Chinese herbology or in Ayurvedic medicine.

Michael Tierra, Herbalist
April, 1986
Santa Cruz, California

The Yoga of Herbs

HERBOLOGY: EAST AND WEST

Herbs, both in the east and the west, have been the prime medicinal agent in traditional and holistic therapies. In the East, particularly India and China, an extensive and intricate herbal science has been developed. Originating from the vision of men of spiritual knowledge, herbal medicine was then refined by thousands of years of experience. In this regard Ayurveda includes what is probably the oldest, most visionary, most developed science of herbal medicine in the world. Such a fully developed system does not need refinement but rather translation and adaptation. This book begins with the effort of conveying the ancient science of Ayurvedic herbalism to our own modern needs.

Some may be of the opinion that the herbal medicine of India is not relevant to us today. Since its system is ancient and traditional, filled with religion and superstition, we may feel it does not apply. Or we may think its herbs are largely from tropical plants that we can have no access to, or which have little value in our climate, our particular environment. At the same time, many of us realize the necessity of incorporating a spiritual/psychological approach with therapy. Just as physical ailments usually follow emotional imbalances, so we may find the spiritual use of herbs in the Indian tradition of particular importance in our own unbalanced society. Far from being out of touch with today's world, Ayurvedic herbal medicine is needed now more than ever.

While some major herbs in Ayurvedic usage have no equivalents in western herbalism, many common western herbs like bayberry, barberry and calamus are also commonly used in India, and Ayurveda contains much useful information about them. Even special Ayurvedic herbs, like *ashwagandha* and *haritaki*, may be incorporated into western herbalism, just as ginseng and tang kuei have come from Chinese sources; just as gotu kola, which originally came from India, is now much in use in this country. Many Ayurvedic herbs are common spices—ginger, turmeric, coriander and fenugreek. An impressive pharmacology of Ayurvedic herbs can be put together merely from herbs and spices commonly available in America.

Ayurveda means "The Science of Life." It does not mean Hindu medicine, nor must its herbalism be considered Indian herbalism. It is a science of living that encompasses the whole of life, and which relates the life of the individual to that of the universe. As such it is open to and includes all life, and all methods that bring us into greater harmony with life.

Ayurveda is not of the east or the west, of ancient or modern time. It is one with all life, a knowledge that belongs to all living beings—not a system imposed upon them, but a resource to be drawn upon freely and to be adapted to the unique needs of the individual in his or her particular environment.

Ayurvedic herbalism gives us not only specific herbs, but a way of understanding all herbs. Ayurveda welcomes the removal of barriers between human beings. The sharing of human healing knowledge must develop for the new age to come. But it must find its place in the immediate world of today. And that is the true purpose of this book.

"The essence of all beings is Earth. The essence of the Earth is
Water. The essence of Water is plants. The essence of plants is the
human being."

*"Esam bhutanam prthivi rasha, prthivya apo raso-pam osadhayo rasa, osad-
hinam puruso rasah."*

Chandogya Upanishad I.1.2.

THE MANIFESTATION OF CONSCIOUSNESS INTO PLANTS

Evolution is a manifestation of latent potentials. Within each thing
is contained all things. In the seed is the tree; in the tree is the forest.
Therefore, intelligence is contained implicitly in the many worlds of
nature, not only in our human-centered world. Another way of saying
this is that consciousness exists in all forms of life. It is the very basis of
creation, the power of evolution. Life, creation, and evolution are the
stages in the unfoldment of consciousness. There is nothing in existence
that is unfeeling, nothing that is profane or unspiritual, nothing without
a unique value in the cosmos. Life is relational, interdependent, intercon-
nective, a system of mutual nourishment and care, not only physically,
but also psychologically and spiritually.

Consciousness, therefore, is not merely thought, much less intellect
or reason. It is the feeling of being alive and being related to all life. Consciousness as pure feeling exists already in the plant and is hidden in the
rock, even within the atom itself. Elemental attraction and repulsion are
similar to love and hate, like and dislike. For this reason, the ancient seers
of India held that the Self alone exists, that unity is the basis of all
existence—that the unity of life is the unity of consciousness.

By this they meant that every living thing was sentient, that every-
thing was, in the sense of consciousness, human. True humanity, which
is humane feeling for all life, is at the heart of all life. Plants and animals
sometimes show this sense of caring more than certain humans, who
have been hardened in their isolated sense of humanity. It is only when
we come to look upon all things as human that we are capable of a truly
humane existence. Such a lesson is taught to us by plants and herbs

whose existence is still grounded in the unity of nature, through which we may return to understand ourselves better.

Man as microcosm contains within himself all the elemental, mineral, vegetable and animal kingdoms. Within the plant is the potential of the human being. Conversely, within the human being is the underlying energy structure of the plant. Our nervous system, it could be said, is a tree whose plant-essence is human. Therefore, plants may communicate directly to that essence of feeling which makes a true human being.

The Plant Kingdom exists to bring feeling into manifestation. On the plant level, feeling exists in a pure and passive form. The animal and human kingdoms manifest this more actively, more separately, but often with less beauty. Consciousness in plants is on a primal level of unity; therefore it is more psychic, telepathic.

Life forms are stations for the reception and transmission of forces, through which all are nourished. Each thing exists to nourish all others, and, in return, to be nourished itself. In this manner each kingdom of nature serves to receive and transmit life. This life is implicit in light and in the transmission of stellar or astral forces.

The earth, like a gigantic receptor or radio-station, inhales and exhales stellar and cosmic forces, the absorbed essence of which grows and unfolds as life. These forces are not all material, but include subtle energies of an occult or spiritual nature. Plants transmit the vital-emotional impulses, the life-force that is hidden in light. That is the gift, the grace, the power of plants.

Plants bring us the love, the nourishing power of the sun, which is the same energy of all the stars, of all light. These cosmic energies emanated by plants thus nourish, sustain and make grow our own astral body. In this way the existence of plants is a great offering, a sacrifice. They offer us not only their own nutritive value but the very light and love from the stars, from the cosmos whose messengers they are. They bring to us the universal light so that we can enter the universal life. They exist for psychological, as well as physical nourishment. Our feelings, then, are our own inner plants, our own inner flowers. They grow in accordance with our perception of the nature of all life.

Creation is light. In the *Vedas*, the ancient scriptures of India, the great god *Agni*, the principle of Fire, the Divine Seer-Will, builds up the worlds, and makes of all creation a series of self-transformations.

Plants exist to transmute light into life. Human beings exist to transmute life into consciousness, love. These three—light, life and love—are one, each an expression of the other, three dimensions of the same existence. Plants transmute light into life through photosynthesis. The human being transmutes life into consciousness through perception. Through direct perception, the seer is the seen, the observer the observed. The Sanskrit word for the plant *osadhi* means literally a receptacle or mind, *dhi*, in which there is burning transformation, *osa*. In the *Vedas* this can mean not only plants but all entities in creation.

The human being is the plant of consciousness. The plant, which effects a similar process on a "lower level" of evolution, feeds our mind and nervous system to help in this process. As below, so above; all the universe is a metamorphosis of light.

In the outer world, a central sun is the source of light and life. In the inner world, a central sun is also the source of life. This inner sun is our true Self, what the ancients called the *Purusha* or *Atman*. Plants bring us into communion with the energy of the outer sun, while our inner plant, our nervous system, brings us into communion with the inner sun. Establishing the proper link between the outer plant and the inner plant thus completes the circuit of light and life, and establishes the free flow of awareness in which the mind is liberated—unites the sun with the sun, merges the outer with the inner, creates a festival of delight in living.

The proper usage of a plant or herb, during which its true power is released, implies a communion with it. The plant, when we are one with it, will vitalize our nervous system and invigorate our perception. This means giving value to a plant as something sacred, as a means of communion with all nature. Each plant, then, like a *mantra*, will help to actualize the potential of cosmic life of which it is a representative.

For this reason, many ancient people have had reverence for the plant kingdom. It is not a superstitious awe, nor a mere sensitivity to beauty, but a reception of the power that plants bring to us. The force is not received simply through ingesting the plant, but in our total communion with it.

The sages of ancient India approached healing and herbs with this same consciousness. Theirs was not a science of experimentation, but a form of direct participation. Experimentation implies distance, a division between observer and observed, subject and object. As a result, it is mediated, measured, translated. In dissecting the corpse, the penetration of the soul is missed. Direct perception, or meditation, is the science of yoga. Yoga allows the essence, the thing-in-itself, to disclose itself. When this happens, a full revelation of material and spiritual potential occurs.

The seers, through the yoga of perception, let plants speak to them. And the plants disclosed their secrets—many of which are far more subtle than a chemical analysis could uncover. Approaching plants in the same way today, not as objects for self-aggrandizement but as integral parts of our own unity, the true value of a plant will flourish for our unselfish use.

To become a true herbalist, therefore, means to become a seer. This means to be sensitive to the being of the herbs, to commune in receptive awareness with the plant-light of the universe. It is to learn to listen when the plant speaks, to speak to the plant as to another human being, and to look upon it as one's teacher.

THE BACKGROUND OF AYURVEDIC MEDICINE

SPIRITUAL BACKGROUND

In order to understand the Ayurvedic approach to herbs, one must understand the basic system of Ayurveda, which is a complete healing science, including the physical, psychological and spiritual aspects of life.

The ancient seers of India envisioned two fundamental principles behind existence: *Purusha*, the Primal Spirit, the principle of sentience of consciousness; and the *Prakruti*, or Great Nature, the principle of creativity. The union of these two, Spirit and Matter, produces all things.

Yet these two are also one, the primordial Two-in-One, Consciousness and its creative, executive force, *Shiva-Shakti*. Within all things is essence, individuality, consciousness—the *Purusha*. Within all things is also the power of manifestation, the capacity for creative enfoldment— *Prakruti*.

From these two great forces in their initial coming together is born Cosmic Intelligence, *Mahat*, which contains the seeds of all manifestation. Inherent in *Mahat* are all the laws of nature.

The Cosmic Intelligence also exists in the human being as the intelligence in the individual. As such it is called *Buddhi*, the means of awakening, developing fully which one becomes enlightened, a *Buddha*. *Buddhi* is our capacity for perception, our ability to discern the real from the unreal.

But this intelligence, in its evolution into material forms, may give rise to the ego, the sense of separate self, or *Ahamkara*. It is the principle of division as it is only our sense of a separate ego that divides us from the unity of life.

In turn, the ego gives rise to the conditioned mind or conditioned consciousness called *Manas*, which, as our sense of self-consciousness, creates a protective thought-field around itself in which we become bound.

Finally, this links us up with the collective unconscious called *Chitta*, the storehouse of thoughts of all limited mentalities. Through *Chitta* we remain under the influence of the latencies, compulsions and drives of the earlier stages of evolution, going all the way back to the animal realm — and before.

Ayurveda aims at a life in harmony with Cosmic Intelligence, whereby our own intelligence is perfected, so that through it we can return to unity with nature; and through nature to our true self and spirit, the *Purusha*. This is the spiritual background of Ayurveda, which is the same as that of yoga, and the basis of Ayurvedic psychology.

This requires the awakening of intelligence wherein we go beyond the rule of the ego. The ego is the basis for all deviation from nature. Health is natural, *Prakruti*. Disease is artificial, *Vikruti*. Hence, most diseases, except those natural to the course of time, are from the psychological imbalance born of unnecessary self-consciousness.

THE THREE *GUNAS*

Prakruti consists of three basic qualities, three prime attributes (called *gunas* in Sanskrit): *Sattva*, the principle of light, perception, intelligence and harmony; *Rajas*, the principle of energy, activity, emotion and turbulence; and *Tamas*, the principle of inertia, darkness, dullness and resistance.

While each of these three qualities is necessary in nature, *Sattva* is the proper quality of the mind. *Rajas* and *Tamas*, in the mind, become impurities that weaken our power of perception.

Individuals in whom *Sattva* predominates give value to truth, honesty, humility and the good of all. Those in whom *Rajas* is strongest value power, prestige, authority and control. Those dominated by *Tamas* remain trapped in fear, servility, ignorance, and the forces of decay.

Hence, it is important to follow a life-style that is predominately *Sattvic*. As these three qualities exist in all nature, it is important to use foods and herbs that are primarily *Sattvic* in nature. In this light, Ayurveda classifies herbs according to the three *gunas*.

This does not mean that herbs of *rajasic* or *tamasic* nature should not be used. As *Sattva* is also the balance of *Rajas* and *Tamas*, *rajasic* herbs may be taken to correct *tamasic* conditions or vice versa. But *sattvic* herbs have value in themselves for promoting the development of the mind.

DIAGRAM 1
COSMIC EVOLUTION

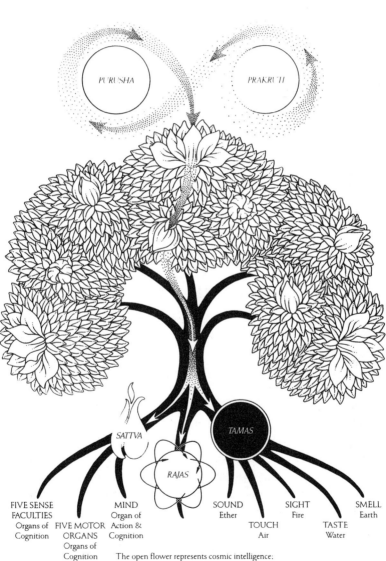

FIVE SENSE · MIND · SOUND · SIGHT · SMELL
FACULTIES · Organ of · Ether · Fire · Earth
Organs of · FIVE MOTOR · Action & · TOUCH · TASTE
Cognition · ORGANS · Cognition · Air · Water
· Organs of
· Cognition · The open flower represents cosmic intelligence;
· the closed flower represents the ego.

THE FIVE ELEMENTS

From the three *Gunas* arise the five elements. From *Sattva*, consisting of clarity, comes the element ether. From *Rajas*, consisting of energy, comes fire. From *Tamas*, consisting of inertia, comes earth. Between *Sattva* and *Rajas* arises the subtle but mobile element air. And between *Rajas* and *Tamas* arises water, combining mobility with inertia.

These elements are the five states of matter: solid, liquid, radiant, gaseous and ethereal. They delineate the five densities of all substances, all visible or invisible matter in the universe. They have psychological correspondences that indicate states of mind and qualities of emotion.

The five parts of plants in Ayurveda, *pancangam*, show how plant structure is related to the five elements. The root corresponds to earth, as the densest and lowest part, connected to the earth. The stem and branches correspond to water, as they convey the water or sap of the plant. The flowers correspond to fire, which manifests light and color. The leaves correspond to air, since through them the wind moves the plant. The fruit corresponds to ether, the subtle essence of the plant. The seed contains all five elements, containing the entire potential plant within itself.

THE THREE *DOSHAS*

At the heart of Ayurveda is its concept of the three *Doshas,* or the three different basic types of human constitution. From ether and air comes *Vata*; from fire and an aspect of water comes *Pitta*; and from water and earth comes *Kapha*. By the elements and *Doshas*, we determine the basic nature of different individuals and we establish a line of treatment unique to their needs.

The three *Doshas* can be recognized by their attributes: *Vata* is dry, cold, light, mobile, subtle, hard, rough, changeable and clear. It is the most powerful of the *Doshas*, being the life-force itself, the strongest to create disease. It governs all movement, and carries both *Pitta* and *Kapha*.

Pitta is hot, light, fluid, subtle, sharp, malodorous, soft and clear. It governs heat, temperature and all chemical reactions. *Kapha* is cold, wet, heavy, slow, dull, static, smooth, dense and cloudy. It maintains substance, weight and coherence in the body.

Vata, in its natural state, maintains energy of will, inhalation, exhalation, movement, the discharge of impulses, equilibrium of the tissues, acuity of the senses. When aggravated, it causes dryness, dark discolorations, desire for warmth, tremors, abdominal distention, constipation, loss of strength, insomnia, loss of sensory acuity, incoherency of speech, and fatigue.

Pitta, in its normal state, is responsible for digestion, heat, visual perception, hunger, thirst, lustre of skin, intelligence, determination, courage, and softness of the body. When aggravated, it causes yellow discoloration of urine, feces, eyes and skin, and may create hunger, thirst, burning sensations and difficulty in sleeping.

Kapha, in its normal state, is responsible for firmness and stability, maintenance of bodily fluids, lubrication of joints, and such positive emotions as peace, love and forgiveness. When aggravated, it produces loss of digestive power, accumulation of phlegm and mucus, exhaustion, feeling of heaviness, pallor, cold sensations, looseness of limbs, difficulty of breathing, coughing and excessive desire for sleeping.

Vata dwells in the colon, hips, thighs, ears, bones and sense of touch. Its main site is the colon where it accumulates, causes disease, and from which it can be expelled directly from the body.

Pitta dwells in the small intestine, stomach, sweat, sebum, blood, plasma, and sense of sight. Its main location is the small intestine where it accumulates, and from which it can be directly expelled from the body.

Kapha dwells in the chest, throat, head, pancreas, ribs, stomach, plasma, fat, nose, and tongue. Its main site is the stomach where it accumulates and causes disease, and from which it can be directly expelled from the body.

Determining Individual Constitution

Individual constitution is acquired at birth and remains constant through life. While there are three general types according to the predominant *Dosha*, combinations and variations also exist. For example, two *Doshas* may exist in equal strengths. The following indications are not to create stereotypes but to just show typical conditions and tendencies towards excess.

VATA

People of *Vata* constitution tend to be physically underdeveloped. Their chests are flat and their veins and muscle tendons are visible. Their complexion is tinged brown, while the skin may be cold, rough, dry or cracked. There usually are a few moles present and these tend to be dark. *Vata* people, in general, are either tall or short, with thin frames that reveal prominent joints due to low muscle development. The hair is most often curly and scanty, with thin eyelashes. The eyes may be small, active, perhaps sunken or lacking in lustre and the conjunctiva is dry and somewhat dark. The nails may be brittle or rough; the nose bent or up-turned.

Physiologically, the appetite and digestion are variable. Sometimes they may be able to consume a large meal with ease, other times they may have no appetite at all. They prefer hot drinks. The production of urine tends to be scanty and the feces are dry, hard, or small in quantity, with a tendency towards constipation. They seldom perspire much. Their sleep may be light, disturbed, or short in duration. Their hands and feet are often cold.

Such individuals are usually creative, active, alert and restless. They talk fast, move and walk quickly but may be easily fatigued or tired.

Psychologically, they are characterized by quick mental understanding, but they are often possessed of a short memory, and can be absent-minded. They adjust easily to change but may become indecisive or impatient. They usually need to develop endurance, confidence and boldness. They may think and worry too much, are often nervous, and it is fear and anxiety that most afflict them.

PITTA

Pitta constitution people are usually of medium height, with moderate weight, frame, and muscle development. Their chests are not as flat as *Vata* people, and they show a moderate number of veins and muscle tendons. They may have many moles or freckles, which are bluish or brownish-red. The bones are not as prominent as in *Vata* types.

Pitta complexion may be coppery, yellowish, reddish or fair. The skin is soft, warm and less wrinkled than *Vata* skin. It possesses good color and may be flushed. The hair is thin, silky, red or brownish and there is a ten-

DIAGRAM 2
SEATS OF VATA, PITTA, KAPHA

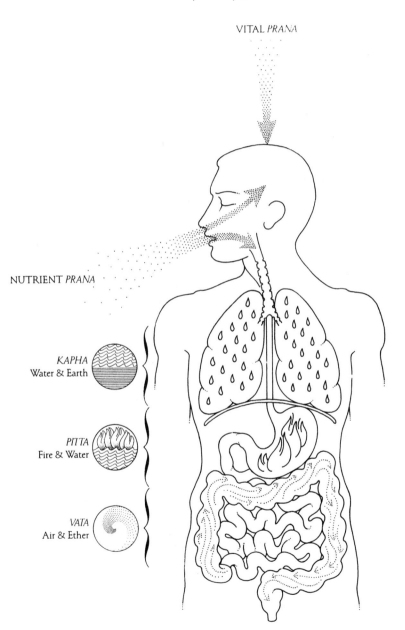

TABLE
THE HUMAN CONSTITUTION (*PRAKRUTI*)

ASPECT OF CONSTITUTION	VATA	PITTA	KAPHA
⚪ Frame	Thin	Moderate	Large
⚪ Body Weight	Low	Moderate	Heavy
⚪ Skin	Dry, Rough, Cool, Brown, Black	Soft, Oily, Warm, Fair, Red, Yellowish	Thick, Oily, Cool, Pale, White
⚪ Hair	Black, Dry, Kinky	Soft, Oily, Yellow, Early Gray, Red	Thick, Oily, Wavy, Dark or Light
⚪ Teeth	Protruded, Spaces Between, Crooked, Gums Emaciated	Moderate in Size, Soft or Bleeding Gums	Strong, White, Full, Well-Formed
⚪ Eyes	Small, Dry, Active, Brown, Black	Sharp, Penetrating, Green, Gray, Yellow	Big, Attractive, Blue, Thick Eyelashes
⚪ Appetite	Variable, Low	Good, Sharp, Excessive	Slow but Steady
⚪ Disease Tendency	Nervous Disorders, Pain	Heat, Infection, Inflammation	Excess Water, Mucus
⚪ Thirst	Variable	Excessive	Slight
⚪ Elimination	Dry, Hard, Constipated	Soft, Oily, Loose	Thick, Oily, Heavy, Slow

Note: *Circles have been provided next to the aspects for those who wish to determine a general idea of individual constitutional make-up. Mark V for Vata, P for Pitta, or K for Kapha in each circle according to the description best fitting each aspect.*

To experience characteristics different from one's respective Dosha might indicate a derangement of that Dosha.

ASPECT OF CONSTITUTION	VATA	PITTA	KAPHA
○ Physical Activity	Very Active	Moderate	Lethargic
○ Mind	Restless, Active Curious	Aggressive, Intelligent	Calm, Slow, Receptive
○ Emotional Excesses	Fearful, Insecure, Anxious	Aggressive, Irritable, Jealous	Greedy, Attached, Self-Contented
○ Faith	Wavering, Changeable	Determined	Steady, Loyal
○ Memory	Recent Memory Good, Remote Memory Poor	Sharp	Slow but Prolonged
○ Dreams	Flying, Jumping, Running, Fearful	Fiery, Angry, Passionate, Colorful	Watery, Ocean, Swimming, Romantic
○ Sleep	Scanty, Interrupted	Little but Sound	Heavy, Prolonged, Excessive
○ Speech	Fast, Chaotic, Uninterrupted	Sharp, Clear, Cutting	Slow, Monotonous, Melodious
○ Spending Habits	Spends Quickly, Impulsively	Spends Moderately & Methodically	Spends Slowly, Saves
○ Pulse	Thready, Feeble, Moves Like a Snake	Moderate, Jumping Like a Frog	Broad, Slow, Moves Like a Swan

Add up all the marks. The Dosha marked most often will generally indicate one's primary constitution. The Dosha marked next frequently will generally indicate the secondary Dosha. It may happen that the two will be relatively equal; that the constitution may be dual (i.e. Vata/Pitta, Vata/Kapha, Pitta/Kapha). Occasionally, all three may be relatively equal and a balanced or Tridosha type may exist.

dency towards early graying or baldness. The eyes may be grey, green or copper-brown. The eyeballs are usually of medium prominence with vision often being poor. The conjunctiva is usually moist and copper-colored, the nails soft; the shape of the nose is sharp and the tip may be reddish.

Physiologically, *Pitta* people possess a strong metabolism, good digestion, and strong appetite. They usually ingest large quantities of food and liquid, and they enjoy cold drinks. Their sleep is of moderate yet uninterrupted duration and the feces are also yellowish, soft and plentiful. They usually perspire a lot. The body temperature is high and the hands and feet are usually warm. They are not easily tolerant of heat or sunlight.

Psychologically, *Pitta* people have good powers of comprehension; they are intelligent and sharp, and can be good orators. They have emotional tendencies of anger, jealousy, perhaps hatred. They are often ambitious and like to be leaders.

KAPHA

Kapha individuals usually have well-developed bodies. However, they tend to carry excess weight. Their chests are expanded and broad; veins and tendons are not obvious because of the thickness of their skin. Their muscle development is good and their bones are not prominent.

Kapha complexion is most often fair, white or pale. Skin tends to be soft, oily, moist, and cold. Hair is thick, dark, soft and wavy. Their eyes are dense, black or blue in color; the white of the eye is usually pronounced, large and attractive. The conjunctiva is seldom reddish.

Physiologically, *Kapha* people have low but regular appetites; their digestion functions slowly, and they usually take less food than other types. They tend to move slowly. Their stools are generally soft and may be pale in color, with slow evacuation. Their perspiration is moderate. Sleep is sound, prolonged, or excessive. They generally have strong endurance and good stamina, and are often healthy and contented.

Psychologically, they tend to be tolerant, calm, forgiving, loving. On the negative side, they are prone to traits of greed, attachment, envy and possessiveness. Their comprehension is slow, yet definitive. Though it takes them time to understand something, their knowledge is retained.

The Three *Doshas* and Plants

The three *Doshas* exist in plants as they do in all nature. *Kapha* plants are characterized by luxuriant growth, abundant leaves and sap; they are dense, heavy, succulent, and contain much water. *Vata* plants have sparse leaves, rough, cracked bark, crooked, gnarled branches, spindly growth habits, and contain little sap. *Pitta* plants are brightly colored with bright flowers; they are moderate in strength and sap, and the latter may be poisonous or burning in its effect.

Soils, climates, geographical zones, and countries can similarly be classified by *Dosha*. Through this we can understand the life-forms produced by them and how to adapt to them.

The root and bark of plants (representing the elements of earth and water) tend to work on *Kapha* conditions. The flowers (as fire) tend to work on *Pitta*. The leaves and fruits (as air and ether) tend to work on *Vata*.

The Three *Doshas* and the Treatment of Disease

To use herbs, or to apply effectively any form of therapy, it is necessary to know the unique constitution of the individual, as well as the specific nature of the disease. Western Medicine, and to some extent, western herbalism, lacks this science of individual constitution.

The same disease may occur in different constitutions, and as such must be treated differently. Asthma, for example, may be due to deranged *Kapha*, excessive water in the lungs; deranged *Vata*, nervous hypersensitivity of the lungs; or deranged *Pitta*, an accumulation of damp-heat in the lungs. The same treatment cannot work in every case. Merely to know that a certain herb "works" on a certain disease may not reveal a definitive cure.

On the other hand, the same constitutional problem, the same aggravated *dosha*, may give rise to various diseases, and as such all can be treated the same way—by decreasing the aggravated *dosha*. High *Vata*, for example, may manifest as sciatic pain, arthritis, constipation, headaches, dry skin, gas and indigestion, all of which can be relieved by a single line of treatment.

Knowing which disease an herb treats gives us one reference line. Knowing the constitution on which it works yields yet another cross reference line. Considering both we are much more able to pinpoint a truly effective treatment.

THE SEVEN *DHATUS* AND *OJAS*

Ayurveda categorizes herbs according to the *dhatus* or tissues upon which they work. It also contains a knowledge of special herbs and substances (minerals and metals) that work on the subtler tissues, including the nerve and reproductive tissues.

The semen or reproductive tissue is the essence of all bodily tissues and contains within itself not only the power of reproduction, but also that of rejuvenation. The essence of the semen, the cream of the body, is called *Ojas*, which means "that which invigorates." *Ojas* is thus the essence of the body, the substance of all hormonal secretions, and supports the auto-immune system.

The plant, like the human being, and the universe itself, is similarly composed of seven *dhatus* or seven planes. The juice of the plant is its plasma. The resin of the plant is its blood. The softwood is muscle. The gum is its fat. The bark is its bones. The leaves are its marrow and nerve-tissue. The flowers and fruit are its reproductive tissue. The flowering tree shows these tissues in their most developed state. The tree is to the plant world what the human being is to the animal kingdom.

The *Dhatus* of the plant work upon the corresponding *Dhatus* of the human body: its juice works upon our plasma; resin upon our blood; softwood upon our muscles; gum upon our fat; bark upon our bones; leaves upon our marrow/nerves; flowers/fruit upon our reproductive organs. The seeds of plants thus treat congenital diseases and dysfunctions by virtue of their affinity with our own seed and congenital root.

Plants similarly possess their own *Ojas*—the energy and love within their system. But, they can transmit *Ojas* when used with love. Remedies produced with love, even when not "therapeutically sound", may work wonders. Love is the true healing force; herbs and other means are merely vehicles.

There are special herbs, like *ashwagandha*, which contain high amounts of *Ojas*, and special ways to prepare herbs which help to transmit them directly. *Mantra* and meditation are part of this process.

We can envision the plant as a human being and the human being as

DIAGRAM 3
THE SEVEN *DHATUS* IN PLANTS

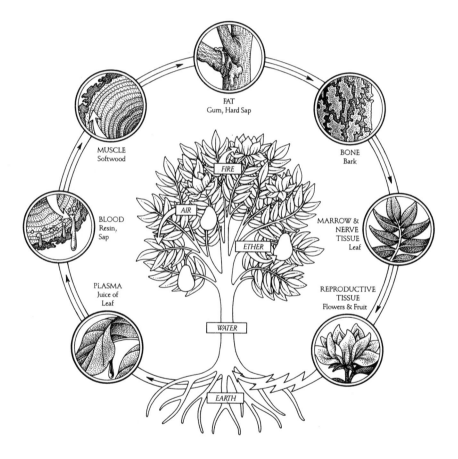

FAT
Gum, Hard Sap

MUSCLE
Softwood

BONE
Bark

BLOOD
Resin,
Sap

MARROW &
NERVE
TISSUE
Leaf

PLASMA
Juice of
Leaf

REPRODUCTIVE
TISSUE
Flowers & Fruit

FIRE

AIR

ETHER

WATER

EARTH

a plant, both composed of the seven *Dhatus.* In this meditation we harmonize the tissues of our body with the great healing powers of nature. Please refer to *AYURVEDA: The Science of Self-Healing,* pages 44-47 for more information.

THE FIVE *PRANAS*

The concept of the life-force is central to all ancient healing traditions, like the concept of Chi in Chinese Medicine. In Ayurveda this life-force, called *Prana,* has five functional variations. Herbs are classified according to which of these *Pranas* they work on.

1. *PRANA:* centered in the brain, it moves downward, governing inhalation and swallowing. It relates to intelligence, power of sensory and motor functions, and primarily to the nervous and respiratory systems.

2. *VYANA:* centered in the heart, it acts throughout the body, governing the circulatory system and the movement of joints and muscles.

3. *SAMANA:* centered in the small intestine, it governs the digestive system.

4. *UDANA:* centered in the throat, it governs speech, energy, will, effort, memory, exhalation.

5. *APANA:* centered in the lower abdomen it governs all downward discharges of feces, urine, semen, menstrual fluid and the fetus.

These five *Pranas* are commonly called the five *Vayus* (*Vayu* means air or motivating force). They are a fivefold division of the life-force and its functional differentiation in its energization of the nervous system.

BODILY SYSTEMS (*SROTAS*)

Ayurveda perceives the human body as composed of innumerable channels. These maintain the metabolism of the various tissues, governing their processes of assimilation and elimination. Disease, then, is an impairment in the flow through these channels: excessive flow, deficient flow, flow in the wrong direction, flow out of the improper channel, blockage of flow.

DIAGRAM 4
THE BREATH IN PLANTS

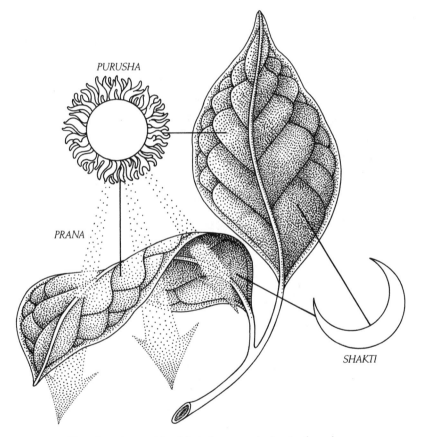

The right and upper sides of the leaf represent the *Purusha*, the male force, and solar energy which is inhalation. The left and lower sides of the leaf represent the *Shakti*, the female force, and lunar energy which is exhalation.

The main factor in disease is blockage of flow through the channels. This can be caused by the biological humours, *Vata*, *Pitta* or *Kapha*, or by toxic accumulations (*Ama*, see page 44). Maintaining the proper flow in the channels is essential to health and to the prevention of disease.

Some of these systems are identical to the systems of western physiology; others are similar to the meridian concept of Chinese medicine. Herbs are classified according to the bodily systems of channels they affect. These are as follows:

1. *Pranavaha srotas*: the channels which carry the breath or *prana*. These are similar to the respiratory system.

2. *Annavaha srotas*: the channels that carry food, which are essentially the same as the digestive system.

3. *Ambuvaha srotas*: the channels which carry water or which regulate the water metabolism, which are another aspect of the digestive system.

These first three systems of channels govern the intake of substances into the body. The next seven supply the seven *Dhatus* or bodily tissues.

4. *Rasavaha srotas*: the channels that carry the plasma portion of the blood and tissue. They are related specifically to the lymphatic system, but also to aspects of the circulatory system.

5. *Raktavaha srotas*: the channels which carry the blood, specifically, the hemoglobin portion of it, also part of the circulatory system.

6. *Mamsavaha srotas*: the channels which supply the muscle tissues or the muscular system.

7. *Medavaha srotas*: the channels that supply the adipose tissue or fat, which govern fat metabolism, the adipose system.

8. *Asthivaha srotas*: the channels which supply the bones, or the skeletal system.

9. *Majjavaha srotas*: the channels which supply the bone marrow, nerve and brain tissue, essentially the nervous system.

10. *Shukravaha srotas*: the channels which govern the semen or the male reproductive system.

The next three systems or channels govern the elimination of waste-materials from the body.

11. *Purishavaha srotas*: the channels which carry the feces, the excretory system.

12. *Mutravaha srotas*: the channels that carry urine or the urinary system.

13. *Svedavaha srotas*: the channels that carry sweat or the sebaceous system.

There are two other systems for the female.

14. *Artavavaha srotas*: the channels which carry the menstruation or the female reproductive system, which has the same place as *Shukravaha srotas* in the male.

15. *Stanyavaha srotas*: the channels which carry milk or lactation, which are another aspect of the female hormonal system.

Finally there is a special system of channels for the mind. These connect mainly to the *Majjavaha srotas*, the nervous system, and also to the reproductive system.

16. *Manovaha srotas*: the channels that supply the mind or carry mental energy, the psychological system.

In our classification of herbs, system function may not be mentioned apart from tissue correspondence. If, for example, we know an herb works on the bones, it is not necessary to mention it having action on the skeletal system.

AGNI AND PLANTS

Ayurveda views the health of the body as the functioning of a biological fire governing metabolism. It is called *agni*. *Agni* is not simply a symbol for the power of digestion. In the broader sense, it is the creative flame that works behind all life, building up the entire universe as a stage by stage unfoldment of itself, which, thereby, contains within itself the key to all transformations.

Agni is present not only in human beings but in all nature. It has a special abode in plants, which contain the *agni* of photosynthesis.

When *agni* is strong, food is digested properly, toxins of various kinds, largely from undigested food particles, (called *ama* in Ayurveda), accumulate and breed disease.

Plants contain *agni*, through which they digest sunlight and produce life. Herbs can transmit their *agni* to us, their capacity to digest and transform, and this may augment our own power of digestion, or give us the capacity to digest substances we normally cannot. The *agni* of plants can feed our *agni*. Through this interconnection, we join ourselves with the cosmic *agni*, the creative force of life and healing.

The *agni* from plants is magnetically attracted by its opposite nature to the negative life-force of the *ama*, or various toxic accumulations in our body. The result is their neutralization and a restoration of harmony.

Herbs can be used to supplement *agni* and thereby restore our auto-immune system. This restores the power of our aura, which is nothing more than the glow of our *agni*.

By their very nature the right herbs and spices can feed *agni*, directly strengthening the basic energy of body-mind, allowing for the right digestion, not only of food but also experience.

HERBAL ENERGETICS

Ayurveda approaches herbs through a science of energetics. The properties of herbs are related systematically according to their taste, elements, heating or cooling effects, effect after digestion and other special potencies they may possess. As distinct from the complexity of chemical analysis, which often loses us in a maze of details, this simple system of energetics clarifies the basic properties of herbs. It gives us a structure in which they can easily be identified and understood. Therefore they can be used for the individual constitution and condition.

This system of herbal energetics is the main factor in the Ayurvedic understanding of herbs. Chinese herbalism has a similar system of taste and energy. The lack of such a system in western herbalism has placed it at a disadvantage.

In this book we try to explain the action of many western herbs according to the energetics of Ayurveda. Hopefully, we may help to close the above-mentioned gap and facilitate herbal usage on an Oriental level of sophistication. Understanding the principles of energetics is essential for treatment.

TASTE (*RASA*)

Ayurveda states that the taste of an herb is not incidental, but is an indication of its properties. Different tastes possess different effects.

Usually we do not connect taste with therapeutic property. With foods we consider taste for enjoyment value. In western herbalism, we note the taste of an herb more as a means of identification rather than as a means of understanding its effects. There is the general recognition that spicy, pungent herbs tend to be heating and stimulating, or that bitter herbs help reduce fever, but this has not become the basis for any classification of herbs by taste.

The Sanskrit word for taste, *rasa*, has many meanings. All of them help us understand the importance of taste in Ayurveda. *Rasa* means "essence." Taste thus indicates the essence of a plant, and so is perhaps the prime factor in understanding its qualities. *Rasa* means "sap," so that the taste of an herb reflects the properties of the sap which invigorates it.

Rasa means "appreciation," "artistic delight," a "musical note." Thus taste communicates feeling, which again is the essence of the plant. Through it the beauty and power of the plant can be perceived. *Rasa* means "circulation," "to feel lively," "to dance," all of which is reflected in the energizing power of taste.

Taste directly affects our nervous system through the *Prana*, the lifeforce in the mouth, which is connected to the *Prana* in the brain. Taste stimulates nerves, awakens mind and senses to make us lively. Thus taste sets our own *rasa* or vital fluid in motion. Through stimulating *Prana*, particularly the gastric nerves, taste affects *agni* and enhances the power of digestion. It is the good taste of food that is necessary to awaken our *agni* for proper digestion.

For this reason, bland food may not be nourishing in spite of its vitamin or mineral content. Without stimulating *agni*, there is no real power of digestion. Ayurvedic medicine has, therefore, always included the science of cooking with the right spices. Together, they are part of the field of Ayurvedic herbal science.

When we are sick, we lose our sense of taste and our appetite. Taste, appetite, and power of digestion are related. Lack of taste indicates fever, disease, low *agni*, high *ama*. To improve *agni* and eliminate disease, it is necessary to improve our sense of taste. This is why spices are such important Ayurvedic herbs. Desire for tasty food indicates hungry *agni* or disease. The problem is that we have perverted our sense of taste with artificial substances.

Taste is the sensory quality that belongs to the element of water. Plants are the life-form belonging to the element of water. Taste thus reflects the energies and elements that operate in a particular herb.

Cloud water originally has no taste, but all tastes are latent in it.These are gathered as it falls, as it passes through the five elements in the atmosphere and takes on their qualities.

Ayurveda recognizes six main tastes: sweet, sour, salty, pungent, bitter and astringent. These derive from five elements; each taste is composed of two elements. Sweet taste is composed of earth and water; sour of earth and fire; salty of water and fire; pungent of fire and air; bitter of air and ether; and astringent of earth and air.

Sweet taste is basically that of sugars and starches. Sour taste is of fermented or acidic things. Salty is of salt and alkalis. Pungent is the same as spicy or acrid, and is often aromatic. Bitter is of bitter herbs like gentian or golden seal. Astringent taste has a constricting quality, as herbs that contain tannin, like oak bark.

Though the six tastes transmit the properties of the five elements, they are all based on the element of water, which manifests them. It is only when the tongue is wet that we recognize taste.

ENERGY (*VIRYA*)

Virya is the energy, potency or power of herbs, designated in Ayurveda as heating or cooling. Herbs through their taste tend to heat the body or cool it and this produces the most basic energizing effect upon the system.

Pungent taste, as is commonly known in hot peppers, chilis, ginger and other hot spices, has a heating effect. Things sour or acid in taste like citrus or products of fermentation like wine, yogurt or pickles, are heating. Fermentation creates combustion which releases heat. Salt is also heating, which we can experience by the burning sensation it produces on cuts or sores.

Sweet taste is cooling, as sugar counteracts burning sensations in the body. Bitter and cold are often synonymous, as in bitter herbs like gentian and golden seal which reduce fever and inflammation. Astringent taste has a constricting effect, which is the action of something cold like ice, as in such astringent substances like alum, oak bark or witch hazel.

Heating herbs cause dizziness, thirst, fatigue, sweating, burning sensations and they speed the power of digestion. They increase *Pitta*, but generally decrease *Vata* and *Kapha*.

Cooling herbs are refreshing, enlivening, and promote tissue firmness. They are calming and clearing to *Pitta* and to the blood, but generally increase *Vata* and *Kapha*.

"Heating or cooling energy" means that these substances contain, respectively, the energies of fire or water (*agni* or *soma*).

Through their energy the six tastes fall into two groups: 1) pungent, sour and salty cause heat and increase *Pitta*; and 2) sweet, astringent and bitter cause cold and decrease *Pitta*. Energy, *virya*, tells us the effect of an herb on *Pitta dosha*.

Pungent is the most heating taste, followed by sour and then salty. Bitter is the most cooling, followed by astringent and then sweet.

Other Twofold Distinctions

Another important twofold distinction of tastes, though not an independent principle like energy, is whether herbs are drying or moistening.

The main quality of *Vata dosha* is dryness, while that of *Kapha* is wetness. Tastes that are drying (bitter, pungent and astringent) increase *Vata* and decrease *Kapha*. Those that are moistening (sweet, salty and sour) increase *Kapha* and decrease *Vata*.

Pungent is the most drying taste, followed by bitter and then astringent. Sweet is the most moistening taste, followed by salty and then sour.

Drying herbs are composed mainly of the element air, while moistening herbs are composed mainly of water. They produce the effects of their element.

Another, but less important, twofold distinction is heavy or light—whether herbs tend to increase lightness or heaviness in the body. This distinction is similar to drying or moistening. Sour taste, owing to its heating potency and its power to increase digestion, tends to be light. Astringent taste, owing to its constricting effect upon the tissues, tends to be heavy.

Sweet is the heaviest taste, followed by salty and then astringent. Bitter is the lightest taste, followed by pungent and then sour. Tastes that are heavy in quality promote weight and firmness in the body. Those light in quality cause loss of weight, but are stronger in stimulating digestion.

VIPAKA, POST-DIGESTIVE EFFECT

The six tastes are reduced to three in their post-digestive effect, *vipaka*. Sweet and salty tastes, have a sweet *vipaka*, sour has a sour *vipaka*, while bitter, astringent and pungent possess a pungent *vipaka*.

These post-digestive effects relate to processes of absorption and elimination; the final outcome of digestion. The first stage of digestion is in the mouth and stomach; moistening, dominated by the sweet taste. The second stage of digestion is in the stomach and small intestine; heating, dominated by the sour or acid taste. The third stage is in the colon; drying, dominated by the pungent taste. These stages again are *Kapha*, *Pitta* and *Vata*, respectively.

Herbs, particularly in the long-term usage, tend to aggravate the *dosha* whose *vipaka* they possess. Sweet and salty substances promote salivary and other *Kapha* secretions. Sour herbs promote stomach acid, bile, and other manifestations of *Pitta*. Bitter, pungent and astringent herbs increase dryness and gas in the colon, thus aggravating *Vata*.

Sweet and sour *vipakas*, owing to their moistening property, allow for easy and comfortable discharge of urine, feces and intestinal gas. Pungent *vipakas*, from their drying property, create difficulty and discomfort in discharge of waste products.

Sweet *vipaka* also promotes the secretion of *Kapha*, including semen and sexual secretions, and allows for comfortable discharge. Sour *vipaka* increases *Pitta* and acid formation in the body, and reduces semen and sexual secretions (though it promotes the other tissue-elements of the body).

Pungent *vipaka* tends to cause gas, constipation and painful urination. It reduces semen and sexual secretions and gives difficulty and discomfort in their discharge.

Sweet and also sour *vipakas* aggravate *Kapha*, while they alleviate *Vata*. Pungent *vipaka* aggravates *Vata*, while it alleviates *Kapha*. Sour *vipaka* aggravates *Pitta* while sweet *vipaka* alleviates it. Pungent *vipaka* tends to aggravate *Pitta* over a period of time.

Post-digestive effect gives us another reference for understanding the effect of herbs, particularly in long term usage. It is a concept unique to Ayurveda.

PRABHAVA, SPECIAL POTENCY

Taste, energy and post-digestive effect are only a general schemata for understanding the properties of herbs. Herbs also possess subtler and more specific qualities that transcend thought and that cannot be placed into a system of energetics. *Prabhava* can be called "the special potency" of the herb. It is its uniqueness, apart from any general rules about it.

Some herbs possess a property at variance with its basic energetics. Basic, for instance, which though classified as heating in energy, helps bring down almost any kind of fever, even those caused by heat. Some herbal properties, like strong purgative action, are also not defined by energetics alone. Other herbs, sharing the same energetics, may differ widely in special potencies; one may be a purgative, while another may not be. All this is *prabhava*.

Prabhava includes the occult properties of plants, their capacity to affect the mind and psyche on a direct and subtle level. The special and thought-transcending power of *mantras* and rituals, and the external use of gemstones to effect inner changes are also *prabhava*. *Prabhava* includes auric action, astral effect, magnetic effect, and radiation. Even some diseases like cancer originate owing to a kind of *prabhava* or special predisposition whose etiology transcends thought and the reasoning of the materialistic mind.

Ayurveda investigates the occult and spiritual effects of substances, and is not limited to any materialistic or chemical-based theory. It understands the value and the limitation of systems, and only uses them as a guide, not as a rigid rule. This spiritual orientation, one could say, is the *prabhava* of Ayurveda, the special power which can be learned from it.

While the *prabhava* of the plants of India is largely known, that of western plants is largely unknown or forgotten. Certainly our American Indians had similar knowledge but lost it during the depredations of the white man. We should apply the science of energetics to western herbs with care and consistency and the belief that exceptions also make the rule.

DESCRIPTION OF THE SIX TASTES
(Quotes from *Charak Samhita* XVI. 43.)

I. Sweet

"The sweet taste (as it is of the same nature as the human body, whose tissues taste sweet), promotes the growth of all bodily tissues and *Ojas*. Aiding in longevity, it is soothing to the five sense organs and the mind, and gives strength and good complexion. Sweet taste alleviates *Pitta, Vata* and the effects of poison. It also relieves thirst and burning sensation and it promotes the health and growth of skin and hair; it is good for the voice and energy.

"Sweet taste is nourishing, vitalizing, gives contentment, adds bulk to the body, creates firmness. It rebuilds weakness, emaciation, and helps those damaged by disease. It is refreshing to the nose, mouth, throat, lips and tongue, and relieves fits and fainting. The favorite of insects, particularly bees and ants, sweet taste is wet, cooling and heavy.

"Yet when used too much by itself or in excess, sweet taste creates obesity, flaccidity, laziness, excessive sleep, heaviness, loss of appetite, weak digestion, abnormal growth of the muscles of the mouth and throat, difficult breathing, cough, difficult urination, intestinal torpor, fever due to cold, abdominal distention, excessive salivation, loss of feeling, loss of voice, goiter, swelling of the lymph glands, legs and neck, accumulations in the bladder and blood vessels, mucoid accretions in the throat and eyes, and other such *Kapha*-caused diseases."

Sweet taste in terms of western herbalism is nutritive, tonic and rejuvenative. It increases semen, milk and nerve tissue, and promotes tissue regeneration internally or externally. It is demulcent and emollient, moistening, softening and soothing.

Sweet Herbs: Sweet taste is found in herbs that contain sugars, starches or mucilage. It includes bland, starchy and pleasant tastes, and may be mixed with less agreeable secondary tastes. It is relatively uncommon. Typical sweet herbs include almonds, comfrey root, dates, fennel, flaxseed, licorice, maidenhair fern, marshmallow, psyllium, raisins, sesame seeds, slippery elm, and Solomon's seal. Sweet taste in herbs can be increased by processing herbs with various forms of raw sugar, honey, or cooking them in milk.

II. Sour

"Sour taste improves the taste of food, enkindles the digestive fire, adds bulk to the body, invigorates, awakens the mind, gives firmness to the senses, increases strength, dispels intestinal gas and flatus, gives contentment to the heart, promotes salivation, aids swallowing, moistening and digestion of food, gives nourishment. It is light, hot and wet.

"Yet when used too much by itself or in excess, sour taste makes the teeth sensitive, causes thirst, blinking of the eyes, goosebumps, liquifies *Kapha*, aggravates *Pitta* and causes a build-up of toxins in the blood. It wastes away the muscles and causes looseness of the body, creates edema in those weak, injured or in convalescence. From its heating property it promotes the maturation and suppuration of sores, wounds, burns, fractures and other injuries. It causes a burning sensation in the throat, chest and heart."

CHART OF THE SIX TASTES

RASA	ELEMENTS	ENERGY	POST-DIGESTIVE EFFECT	WET/DRY	HEAVY/LIGHT
Sweet	Earth and Water	Cooling – 3	Sweet	Wet – 1	Heavy – 1
Salty	Water and Fire	Heating – 3	Sweet	Wet – 2	Heavy – 2
Sour (Acid)	Earth and Fire	Heating – 2	Sour	Wet – 3	Light – 3
Astringent	Earth and Air	Cooling – 2	Pungent	Dry – 3	Heavy – 3
Pungent	Air and Fire	Heating – 1	Pungent	Dry – 1	Light – 2
Bitter	Air and Ether	Cooling – 1	Pungent	Dry – 2	Light – 1

1 – first degree, strongest action
2 – second degree, moderate action
3 – third degree, least action

Sour taste in terms of western herbalism is stimulant, promotes digestion, increases appetite and is carminative (helps dispel flatus). It is
nourishing to all tissue-elements except reproductive tissue (*shukra dhatu*).
It promotes metabolism, circulation, along with sensory and brain
functioning.

Sour Herbs: Sour taste occurs largely from the presence of various
acids in plants, like acid fruit. Sour taste is rarer than sweet. Typical sour
herbs include hawthorn berries, lemon, lime, raspberries and rose
hips. Sour taste in herbs can be increased by preparing herbs in fermentation as herbal wines or as tinctures in alcohol (whose taste is sour).

III. Salty

"Salty taste promotes digestion, is moistening, enkindles digestive
fire; it is cutting, biting, sharp, fluid. It works as a sedative, laxative,
deobstruent. Salty taste alleviates *Vata*, relieves stiffness, contractions,
softens accumulations, and nullifies all other tastes. It promotes salivation, liquifies *Kapha*, cleanses the vessels, softens all the organs of the
body, gives taste to food. It is heavy, oily and hot.

"Yet when used too much by itself or in excess it aggravates *Pitta*,
causes stagnation of blood, creates thirst, fainting and the sensation of
burning, erosion and wasting of muscles. It aggravates infectious skin
conditions, causes symptoms of poisoning, causes tumors to break
open, makes the teeth fall, decreases virility, obstructs the functioning
of the senses, causes wrinkling of the skin, greying and falling of the
hair. Salty taste promotes bleeding diseases, hyperacidity of digestion,
inflammatory skin diseases, gout and other mainly *Pitta* diseases."

Salty taste in small doses promotes digestion and increases appetite;
in moderate doses functions as a laxative or purgative; and in large doses
is an emetic, promotes vomiting. It is demulcent, softening bodily tissues
and it is calming, mildly sedative. It aids in tissue growth throughout the
body and promotes water retention.

Salty Herbs: Salty taste is really not a plant but a mineral taste, so it
is very rare in plants as a primary taste. Typical salty substances include
epsom salt, Irish moss, kelp, rock salt, sea salt and seaweed. Salty taste in
herbs can be increased by adding salt to herbal preparations.

IV. Pungent

"The pungent taste is cleansing to the mouth, enkindles digestive fire, purifies food, promotes nasal secretions, causes tears and gives clarity to the senses. It helps cure diseases of intestinal torpor, obesity, abdominal swelling and excessive liquid in the body. It helps discharge oily, sweaty and sticky waste products. It gives taste to food, stops itching, helps the resolution of skin growths, kills worms, is germicidal, corrodes the muscle tissues, moves blood clots and blood stagnation, breaks up obstructions, opens the vessels, alleviates *Kapha*. It is light, hot and dry.

"Yet when used too much by itself or in excess causes a weakening of virility by its post-digestive effect. By its taste and hot potency, it causes delusion, weariness, languor, emaciation. Pungent taste causes fainting, prostration, loss of consciousness and dizziness. It burns the throat, generates a burning sensation in the body, diminishes strength and causes thirst. By its predominance of fire and air, pungent taste creates various burning sensations, tremors, and piercing and stabbing pains throughout the body."

Pungent taste is stimulating, promotes digestion, increases appetite, is diaphoretic (causes sweating) and expectorant (removes phlegm) and is vermicidal (kills parasites). It promotes circulation and generally increases all bodily functions, while reducing all foreign accretions in the body.

Pungent Herbs: Pungent taste arises mainly from various aromatic oils. It is more common than sweet but not abundant. Still, many herbs belong to this category and they are very useful and often become spices and condiments. Pungent taste includes acrid, spicy and aromatic.

Typical pungent herbs include angelica, asafoetida, basil, bayberry, bay leaves, black pepper, camphor, cardamom, cayenne, cinnamon, cloves, coriander, cumin, ephedra, eucalyptus, garlic, ginger, horseradish, mustard, onions, oregano, peppermint, prickly ash, rosemary, sage, sassafras, spearmint, thyme, and valerian.

V. Bitter

"Bitter taste, though it does not taste good in itself, restores the sense of taste. It is detoxifying, antibacterial, germicidal, and kills worms. It relieves fainting, burning sensation, itch, inflammatory skin conditions and thirst. Bitter taste creates tightness of the skin and muscles. It is antipyretic, febrifuge; it enkindles digestive fire, promotes digestion of toxins, purifies lactation, helps scrape away fat and remove toxic accumulations in fat, marrow, lymph, sweat, urine, excrement, *Pitta* and *Kapha*. It is dry, cold and light.

> "Yet when used by itself or in excess, owing to its natural properties of dryness, roughness and clearness, it causes a wasting away of all the tissue elements of the body. Bitter taste produces roughness in the vessels, takes away strength, causes emaciation, weariness, delusion, dizziness, dryness of the mouth and other diseases of *Vata*."

Bitter taste reduces fevers, is anti-inflammatory, antibacterial, detoxifying and germicidal. It is cleansing to the blood and all tissues in general and helps reduce tumors. It has a reducing, depleting and sedating effect upon the body, although in small amounts it is stimulating, particularly to digestion.

Bitter Herbs: Bitter is a very common taste in herbs and plants. It arises from various bitter principles like berberine. Bitters may be simple, like gentian. They may be aromatic (pungent secondarily), like wormwood. Or they may be astringent (secondarily) like golden seal.

Typical bitter herbs include aloe, barberry, blessed thistle, blue flag, chapparal, chrysanthemum, dandelion, echinacea, gentian, golden seal, pao d'arco, Peruvian bark, rhubarb, rue, tansy, white poplar, yarrow and yellow dock.

VI. Astringent

> "Astringent taste is a sedative, stops diarrhea, aids in healing of joints, promotes the closing and healing of sores and wounds. It is drying, firming, contracting. It alleviates *Kapha*, *Pitta* and stops bleeding. Astringent taste promotes absorption of bodily fluids; it is dry, cooling and light.
> "Yet when used too much by itself or in excess, it causes drying of the mouth, produces pain in the heart, causes constipation, weakens the voice, obstructs channels of circulation, makes the skin dark, weakens vitality, causes premature aging. Astringent taste causes the retention of gas, urine and feces, creates emaciation, weariness, thirst and stiffness. Owing to its natural properties of roughness, dryness and clearness, it causes *Vata*-diseases like paralysis, spasms and convulsions."

Astringent taste is hemostatic (stops bleeding), stops sweating, stops diarrhea, as it promotes absorption of fluids and inhibits their elimination. It is anti-inflammatory, vulnerary (closes wounds and promotes healing by knitting the membranes back together). It constricts the muscles and helps raise prolapsed organs.

Astringent Herbs: Astringent taste is also very common in herbs, but it is not of such therapeutic importance, as astringent action is used mainly symptomatically. Astringency derives mainly from the presence of various tannins.

Typical astringent herbs include cranesbill, lotus seeds, mullein, plantain, pomegranate, raspberry leaves, sumach, uva ursi, white pond lily, white oak bark and witch hazel.

Combined Tastes

Tastes of herbs are seldom single, though one usually predominates.

Sweet and pungent tastes sometimes combine, as with cinnamon, fennel, ginger and onion. Such herbs are particularly good for *Vata*.

Sweet and astringent often combine, as with comfrey, lotus, slippery elm and white pond lily. Such herbs are particularly good for *Pitta* but may be hard to digest.

Sweet and bitter sometimes combine, as with licorice. These herbs are also particularly good for *Pitta*.

Sweet and sour combine in various fruit like hawthorn and oranges. They are very good for *Vata*.

Pungent and bitter sometimes combine as with motherwort, mugwort, wormwood and yarrow. Such herbs have a strong effect on *Kapha*.

Pungent and astringent combine occasionally, as with bayberry, cinnamon or sage. They also work on *Kapha*.

Bitter and astringent often combine, as in many diuretics. Such herbs include golden seal, plantain and uva ursi. They work mainly on *Pitta*.

Some herbs possess three or more tastes. For herbs of multiple tastes the energy and post-digestive effect become important for determining their effect. Herbs of multiple tastes often possess powerful or broad spectrum healing action like garlic.

Tastes and Foods

Like herbs, foods have therapeutic properties according to the tastes and elements which dominate them. In Ayurveda a special diet is prescribed along with the use of particular herbs. Generally, the patient is told to follow the diet that tends to alleviate his or her particular *Dosha*. However, particular foods are prescribed therapeutically as herbs, or in combination with herbs. Such substances include milk, honey, *ghee*, raisins, dates and almonds. Herbology and nutrition are a single science in Ayurveda, and no treatment can be truly efficacious that neglects one or the other. Food deals with the "grosser nutrition" of the body; herbs give subtle nutrition and stimulation to the deeper tissues and organs.

Tastes and Emotions

Emotions also have a certain taste or flavor and affect the body according to their qualities. There are bitter emotions like grief, or astringent emotions like fear—these aggravate *Vata*. There are sour emotions like envy, or pungent emotions like anger—these aggravate *Pitta*. And there are sweet emotions like desire, or salty emotions like greed—these aggravate *Kapha*.

Emotions can have the same effect upon the body as wrong foods, drugs, alcohol, or infections. Psychological factors have the power to overcome physiological factors in treatment. For this reason Ayurveda also has a science of the energetics of the psyche. The unified body-mind science of Ayurveda allows us to use herbs to help counteract mental states and emotional problems.

The science of *rasa*, or taste, and its energetics, comprehends not only herbs and food but also the mind. Like other aspects of the Ayurvedic language of healing, taste has value on all levels of manifestation, both inner and outer.

MANAGEMENT OF
INDIVIDUAL CONSTITUTION (*DOSHA*)

In Ayurveda, patients are treated according to their constitution. The treatment is not symptomatic, but goes to the root of the individual's physiological and psychological being. The purpose of Ayurveda is not to cure a particular disease, but to bring each individual to his or her own natural self-harmony. This goes to the heart of all diseases that are manifested in the individual. In treating the "disease" the healer is only working generally or superficially.

Knowledge of constitution is the key for a holistic and integral health care, the true basis of any preventive medicine. In differentiating diseases according to constitution, we understand why different herbs treat the same disease or why certain herbs treat many diseases.

In Ayurveda we treat the individual constitution by its predominate *Dosha*. Generally speaking, we treat the *Dosha* with herbs and therapies of an opposite nature to its qualities. Heating and drying therapies are used for *Kapha* constitution which tends towards cold and dampness. Heating and moistening are used for *Vata* that tends towards cold and dryness; and cooling and drying is used for *Pitta* whose properties are hot and moist.

However, sometimes herbs that increase a particular *Dosha* may help in treating it. Some herbs that increase *Kapha*, like licorice, in liquifying excess or accumulated *Kapha* by the moistening effect of the herb, facilitate its elimination from the body. Hence because an herb may increase a particular *Dosha* does not mean that such an herb can never be used to treat that *Dosha*. It may be helpful for short term usage or as balanced out by other herbs more opposite to the *Dosha* in properties. Herbal therapies and formulas must be examined as a whole, according to their complete strategy and final outcome.

Individual Constitution and Disease Condition

Individual constitution generally represents the disease-proneness of the individual; for example, *Kapha* people tend to suffer from *Kapha*-type diseases like colds and congestive disorders. However, individuals can also

suffer from diseases of a different nature than their constitution, like a
Kapha-type common cold suffered by a *Pitta* person. So we must note not
only the nature of the individual but also that of the disease and treat
both.

Individual constitution is called *Prakruti* in Sanskrit, which means
"nature." Disease condition is called *Vikruti*, which means "deviation from
nature." Ascertaining an individual's constitution depends more on innate
factors like the build of the body, or on lifelong tendencies and appetites.
Ascertaining the disease condition relates more to symptoms, which may
be temporary.

As long as our herbal treatment deals mainly with acute, temporary
or surface conditions then determination of individual constitution is not
that important. We can more simply and directly treat the disease condition. But for deeper and more chronic diseases, for long term treatment,
knowledge of the constitution is essential for a complete and effective
therapy.

Disease conditions of a different nature than that of the individual are
relatively easy to treat. Those of the same nature are difficult, as the
nature of the individual reinforces the nature of the disease.

MANAGEMENT OF *KAPHA*

Kapha, in which the element of water predominates, is cold, moist,
slow and heavy in attribute. Therefore, it is treated by a warming, drying,
lightening and stimulating therapy. Tastes that treat *Kapha* are pungent,
bitter and astringent; they are all drying and lightening, catabolic in their
actions. Pungent taste, which is also heating, is exactly opposite *Kapha* in
its qualities, and so is most specifically prescribed in treating *Kapha*
conditions.

Therapies that treat *Kapha* are reducing therapies. They are usually
given along with fasting or a light diet. Their action is to reduce weight,
the earth element in the body, and to dispel water.

Water can be eliminated from the body in various ways. The most
direct way is through the kidneys, via urination, in diuresis. Hence, the
diuretic method of therapy, increasing kidney function, is a major anti-
Kapha therapy. It helps dispel edema, water stagnation in the body, and
helps reduce fat, which is also usually an excess of water. Diuretic herbs,
however, do not go to the root of *Kapha* disorders. *Kapha's* main site of

accumulation is in the lungs and stomach, which diuretics working on the kidneys may not directly affect.

Water can also be eliminated from the skin through sweating. Diaphoretic herbs promote sweating and thereby dispel excess *Kapha* through the skin. Sweating is another major anti-*Kapha* therapy. It is effective in dispelling common colds and flus, which are generally a *Kapha* condition, and it also works to dispel water from the surface, beneath the skin, the face and the upper portions of the body. It is useful in the initial stages of febrile diseases, asthma, bronchitis, lymphatic congestion.

Water also exists in the body as phlegm or mucus, which is the basic form of *Kapha* in the body. This can accumulate in the lungs and stomach, and spread to various other parts of the gastrointestinal tract. Water may also go under the skin, and create various tumors, generally benign. Phlegm can lodge anywhere in the body and block the channels of circulation, *srotas*, and create various diseases, like heart disease owing to high cholesterol. To dispel *Kapha* in the form of phlegm and mucus, expectorant or mucus dispelling herbs are used.

According to Ayurveda, the strongest way to reduce *Kapha* is by using emetic therapy. *Kapha* exists primarily in the lungs and stomach, and from there it can best be expelled from the body by therapeutic vomiting. This is an extension of the diaphoretic and expectorant method. *Kapha*, whose energy is sinking, is dispelled by upward moving and dispersing action.

Yet, to be effective, therapeutic vomiting must be done with the right preparations and conditions. It should only be administered by those who have special knowledge or training in this therapy. Vomiting induced at the wrong time, or to the wrong constitution, can severely aggravate the body and the nerves.

Kapha is cold and heavy, the opposite qualities of *Agni*, and so it reduces or suppresses the digestive fire. It is this weakness of the digestive fire (the fire element) that creates the increase of water (*Kapha*), which leads to various diseases.

In this regard, herbs which promote digestion, stimulant and carminative herbs, are another major anti-*Kapha* therapy. They are basically hot, pungent herbs that strengthen *Agni*, increase metabolism, circulation, and promote activity that breaks up the inertia of *Kapha*. This is why spices are good for *Kapha* constitution.

Bitter herbs, particularly those called bitter tonics, are the strongest herbs to reduce fat in the body and thereby also serve strongly to decrease *Kapha*. Bitter herbs are composed mainly of air and so they bring about weight reduction, the decrease of the earth element in the body, which is also *Kapha*. Bitter herbs reduce craving for sweets and promote spleen-pancreas function.

Laxative and purgative herbs, herbs which promote evacuation, may similarly help reduce the earth element in the body and so reduce *Kapha* (though they should be used only where conditions warrant it).

Astringent herbs by their drying, and often diuretic or expectorant action, also have value in reducing *Kapha*.

Many of these herbal therapeutics are related: Many hot, pungent herbs like ginger, cinnamon and cloves possess not only stimulant and carminative actions, but also diaphoretic and expectorant ones. Most hot stimulants possess expectorant action and some possess diaphoretic action. Most diaphoretics are also expectorants. It is the same principle at work; increase fire, reduce water.

Herbal medicine is a most effective therapy in reducing *Kapha*. This is because the predominant tastes of herbs are bitter, astringent and pungent, the three tastes that reduce *Kapha*. Very few herbs increase *Kapha*. Even sweet, tonic and demulcent herbs may be useful in liquifying *Kapha* to aid in its expulsion from the body. Herbs are a good basis for the lightening, reducing and detoxifying therapy used to treat *Kapha*.

MANAGEMENT OF *PITTA*

Pitta, which mainly consists of the element of fire, is primarily hot in attribute. Therefore, it is treated with a cooling or heat-dispelling therapy. It is also moist, light and mobile, so it can benefit from therapies which are drying, nutritive or calming. The cooling therapy, however, should be given first whenever *Pitta* is to be treated.

Tastes that treat *Pitta* are sweet, astringent and bitter—all cooling in nature. Bitter taste, being the coldest and most drying of the tastes, is strongest in reducing *Pitta*.

The treatment of *Pitta* is intimately associated with treatment of the blood, *Rakta*, the tissue-element of the body that relates to *Pitta*. In heat-dispelling therapies, the blood is usually cooled along with *Pitta*. Most problems of blood heat, toxicity and bleeding relate to *Pitta*.

Most conditions of bodily heat, fever, inflammation, infection or acidity also relate generally to *Pitta*. When deranged, *Pitta* will manifest itself in the above aberrations. But *Pitta* or *Agni* may be obstructed or moved by *Vata* and *Kapha*. This gives heat symptoms like fever, but they must be treated by alleviating the *Dosha* causing the problem. We cannot simplistically treat all heat as *Pitta*.

Heat may be dispelled from the body in various ways. We must determine the nature, depth and location of its manifestation to discover the appropriate treatment for it.

Surface heat, as in fever due to colds or temporary (not necessarily chronic or deep-seated) inflammatory skin conditions, is usually treated using diaphoretic herbs. Warming diaphoretics increase heat and cause sweating, thereby aggravating *Pitta*. But there is also a class of cooling diaphoretics that dispel heat and eliminate *Pitta* through sweating. For surface heat due to *Pitta*, *Pitta*-colds etc., these are appropriate.

Heat in the blood, which is found in many inflammatory and infectious conditions, sores, ulcers, boils, infections, etc., can be treated with alterative herbs. These are usually bitter or astringent anti-*Pitta* herbs, often possessing antibacterial properties and promoting healing. Where blood heat leads to bleeding, as is its tendency, astringent or hemostatic herbs can be used, those whose taste and energy alleviate *Pitta*.

For the highest heat, fever and *Pitta*-conditions, bitter fire-purging and heat-dispelling herbs are used. In western herbalism these are called bitter tonics. They are the strongest herbs for cooling *Pitta*, for sedating and detoxifying the liver, and for reducing deep-seated heat/fever in the interior of the body. Ayurveda calls them febrifuges or antipyretic herbs, and advises the use of bitter taste for bringing down fevers. Their action is similar to alteratives but they are stronger, reaching deeper tissues than blood and lymph.

Purgatives, herbs which promote excretion, those whose energy is cooling, are another strong anti-*Pitta* therapy. When the heat attribute of *Pitta* is high, or where there is high fever, this heat accumulates in the gastrointestinal tract and dries up the stool causing constipation. Then purgation can directly alleviate *Pitta*, and it is in this condition that the strongest purgatives tend to be used.

When, however, the liquid attribute of *Pitta* is high, which is generally more common, there is diarrhea or loose motion of a heat nature. In this instance, such cooling purgatives may still be used, as the cause again is heat.

Ayurveda considers the purgative method (*virechana karma*) to be the strongest for eliminating excess *Pitta* from the body, as it clears *Pitta* from its site of accumulation in the small intestine. It is the natural course for the elimination of *Pitta*, but again may require supervision, as it is a strong therapy.

Usually heat is dispelled downwards from the body. Heat rises and expands and so it is dispelled by a sinking and contracting action. For this reason, not only purgative action but also diuretic action, is also helpful for relieving *Pitta*. Urination not only clears water, but heat and acidity from the body, and it also has a strong anti-*Pitta* action.

Pitta often manifests in excessive sweating, diarrhea, bleeding, inflamed ulcerated skin or membranes. For checking these excessive discharges and for promoting healing of ulcerative sores, astringent action herbs can be applied in treating *Pitta* conditions.

When *Pitta*, owing to an excess of liquid attribute, suppresses the digestive fire and leads to indigestion and the build-up of toxins, even some pungent herbs, like ginger, can be used for their stimulating digestive action. But they should be used with care, moderation, or in balance with other herbs. Bitter tonics also help increase *Agni* by their drying action; in addition they do not aggravate *Pitta*.

MANAGEMENT OF *VATA*

Vata, which consists mainly of the element air, is basically cold, dry, light and mobile in attribute. Therefore, it is treated by a therapy which is warming, moistening and promotes weight. Such therapy should also calm hyperactivity. Tastes that decrease *Vata* are sweet, sour, salty; they are all moistening and nutritive in action.

However, many pungent herbs can decrease *Vata*. In fact, a majority of pungent herbs may be used in this way, including some of the strongest anti-*Vata* herbs. Pungent taste only aggravates *Vata* when used in excess.

In this regard, we must distinguish between two general different kinds of *Vata* derangement. These can be referred to as "*Vata*-caused deficiency" ("deficient *Vata*" for short) and "obstructive-*Vata*." "*Vata*-caused deficiency" (*Dhatu-kshaya*) refers to the depletion of tissue through *Vata's* drying and lightening action. Most cases of emaciation, dehydration and deficiency of vital fluids are this kind of *Vata* problem. "Obstructive-*vata*" refers to *Vata* derangement caused by blockage of the channels (*margavarodha*) by accumulated *Vata*, which may also gather with it *Ama*, *Kapha* or *Pitta*. This includes such diseases as arthritis and rheumatism as well as many digestive problems of abdominal distention, gas and constipation. Such accumulated *Vata* may result in obesity or what is called "anabolic *Vata.*"

Vata-caused deficiency is treated with a tonic therapy of mainly sweet and nutritive herbs and foods. In obstructed *Vata* we must remove the obstruction and in this a tonic therapy does not work. A tonic therapy would only feed the obstruction and increase the stagnation of *Vata* causing more pain and discomfort. Hence we use pungent herbs to clear out the obstruction and so alleviate *Vata*.

Pungent taste has a stimulating effect on *Vata* and can thereby help move and dispel accumulated and stagnant *Vata*. This, in the short term, reduces *Vata*; but in the long term, after the blockage in the movement of *Vata* is removed, it will tend to increase *Vata*.

Pungent taste is the hottest taste. It is useful in helping to dispel the cold attribute of *Vata*. It aggravates *Vata* only in terms of dryness. When cold is the main *Vata* attribute to be combatted, we can use pungent taste. When dryness and dehydration are pronounced, it is generally contraindicated.

In the weak or variable digestion characteristic of *Vata*-constitution, pungent herbs are also helpful. As the strongest herbs for promoting *Agni* and destroying toxins, they counter high-*Vata* indigestion and poor assimilation.

In terms of western herbology the following herbs and therapies can be used to alleviate *Vata*: diaphoretics of a warming nature can be used to dispel *Vata* related colds and flus (it is wind that carries the cold into the body). Diaphoretics are also helpful in moistening the skin in the various skin dryness problems that come through *Vata*. These must be used with moderation to not dry *Vata* out further through too much sweating. They are used mainly for obstructed *Vata*. Many possess antirheumatic properties and are useful in arthritis (*Ama Vata*).

Carminative herbs, herbs that dispel gas from the gastrointestinal tract, are used mainly for obstructed *Vata*. Nervine and antispasmodic herbs, herbs that help relieve muscle tension, stop spasms and nervous tremors, are also therapeutic for obstructed *Vata*.

Laxative and purgative therapies are used to dispel the constipation that so often goes with a *Vata* condition. They are used mainly for obstructed *Vata*, but they can greatly aggravate *Vata* if over-used. Laxatives which are moistening and increase bulk, like flaxseed or psyllium seeds, are better for deficient *Vata*. Strong purgatives, such as rhubarb or senna, may be necessary on a temporary basis in dealing with obstructed *Vata*. But they must be used with care.

Stimulant therapies that promote digestion, appetite and the neutralization of *Ama* are very helpful in *Vata* conditions. In obstructed *Vata* they remove blockages of *Ama* and *Kapha*. In deficient *Vata* they promote the appetite and digestion to help rebuild the body.

Deficient *Vata* is treated using tonic, nutritive and rejuvenative herbal therapy and diet. Bitter tonics of western herbology, as they possess the same attributes of *Vata*, are contraindicated. Sweet demulcent and emollient herbs like licorice, slippery elm and comfrey root are the closest to tonic, nutritive herbs in the Ayurvedic sense.

Ayurveda considers enema therapy (*basti*) to be the strongest therapy for eliminating excess *Vata* from the body and thereby getting to the root of all *Vata* disorders. In this treatment, various medicated herbal and oil enemas are prepared under knowledgeable administration.

Ayurvedic formulas to reduce *Vata* often contain salt, particularly rock salt, which is lighter than sea salt, and a very good digestive stimulant for *Vata*-types.

DETOXIFICATION/MANAGEMENT OF *AMA*

Ama, the accumulation of toxins, undigested food or waste-materials, complicates the treatment of the three *Doshas*. In general, *Ama* possesses the same characteristics as *Kapha*; it is heavy, dense, cold and slimy, consisting largely of mucoid accretions. Yet it can be aligned with any of the *Doshas*.

Doshas aligned with *Ama* are called *"Sama"* (*"sa"* means "with" and combined with *"ama"* becomes *"Sama"* in Sanskrit). *Vata* can accumulate as gas in the large intestine and spread to the small intestine, blocking the power of digestion, *Agni*, and give rise to *Ama*. *Kapha* can accumulate in the stomach as mucus, spread into the small intestine, block *Agni* and also create *Ama*. *Pitta* can accumulate as bile in the small intestine, which though hot, can block *Agni* by its liquidity or oiliness, which similarly gives rise to *Ama*. Such conditions are called respectively *Sama Vata, Sama Kapha* and *Sama Pitta*.

Ama and *Agni* are opposite in properties. *Ama* is cold, wet, heavy, cloudy, malodorous and impure. *Agni* is hot, dry, light, clear, fragrant (aromatic) and pure. To treat *Ama*, it is necessary to increase *Agni*.

Psychologically, *Ama* arises from the holding of negative emotions. Negative emotions quench the mental *Agni* or clarity of mind. As a result, the physical *Agni* is also reduced. Undigested experiences become toxic like undigested food.

Symptoms of *Ama* include loss of taste and appetite, indigestion, tongue-coating, bad breath, loss of strength, heaviness, lethargy, and obstructions of channels and vessels. Other symptoms are accumulation of waste-materials, bad odor of body, urine or feces, deep, heavy or dull pulse, lack of attention, loss of clarity, depression, irritability and obstruction of other *Doshas*.

Ama is the root of most colds, fevers and flus, as well as the chronic diseases of a weak auto-immune system—these range from allergies and hay fever to asthma, arthritis and cancer.

Wherever there is such evidence of *Ama*, treatment must first aim at its elimination. It is not possible to treat two *Dosha*s simply and directly when they are mixed with *Ama*. For example, tonification and rejuvenation therapies are only possible once the body is cleared of *Ama*.

Ama is decreased by herbs that are bitter or pungent in taste. Bitter taste, composed of air and ether, helps separate *Ama*, whose quality is heavy, from the tissues and organs wherein it is lodged. It catalyzes and thereby relieves the fever due to this invasion of *Ama* into the tissues. It stimulates the catabolic processes of the body wherein foreign material is broken down. Like dry ice, it can help destroy *Ama*.

Pungent taste, composed of fire and air, burns up and eradicates *Ama*. It has the same properties as *Agni*, and through strengthening *Agni*, it digests *Ama*. Usually bitter taste is used first to halt the development of *Ama*. Then pungent taste is used to revive the metabolism to consume the *Ama* and prevent it from redeveloping. Bitter taste by itself may not be sufficient to completely destroy Ama or adequately restore *Agni*.

Ama is increased by substances that are sweet, salty or sour in taste. Sweet taste, like *Ama*, is cold, heavy and wet. Salty taste is also heavy and wet. Salty and sour tastes by their hot and damp properties can aggravate the fever and toxic heat of the blood that usually accompanies *Ama*.

Astringent taste is mixed in its action on *Ama*. Its constricting effect upon the tissues and discharges may serve to hold *Ama* in the body. Yet it can be used to help in the healing of membranes damaged by infections due to *Ama*. So it must be used as a supplement to bitter or pungent therapies.

As the main attribute of *Ama* is heaviness, it is treated primarily by herbs and diet of a light nature. Often a fast is a good idea until the tongue clears or the appetite returns. *Ama* as a primary factor in disease is behind the value and extensive usage of fasting, mucus-free diets and detoxifying therapies for many different diseases. Such therapies may have benefit even when the exact constitution of the individual is not determined.

Because the properties of the *Dosha* are mixed with those of *Ama*, herbs which may relieve a *Dosha* may not be effective in a *Sama* condition. Conversely, herbs which normally aggravate a *Dosha* may relieve it in a *Sama* condition. We must discriminate not only the *Dosha* but whether it is with or without *Ama* (*Sama* or *Nirama*, "*nir*" means "without").

Vata, which is normally light and dry, becomes heavy and damp when mixed with *Ama*. *Pitta*, which is hot and damp, becomes cooler and more wet. *Kapha* becomes heavier, and while normally slow in motion, may become stuck or immobile by *Ama*. The turbidity, stickiness and density of *Ama* alters the attributes of the *Doshas*.

> **VATA, SAMA**: Indications: constipation, foul breath and feces, tongue coating, abdominal pain and distention (aggravated by palpation, massage or oil), intestinal gas and cramping pain, low appetite, heaviness, weakness, slow pulse, aggravated by cloudy weather.
>
> Treatment: mainly pungent tasting herbs, stimulants and carminatives, along with some laxatives or purgatives to clear toxins.
>
> **VATA, NIRAMA**: Indications: no constipation, no foul smell, pain mild (relieved by touch), tongue clear, mouth dry with astringent taste, body light, dry, with more emaciation, more tissue depletion, less fatigue.

DIAGRAM 5
MANDALA OF TIME

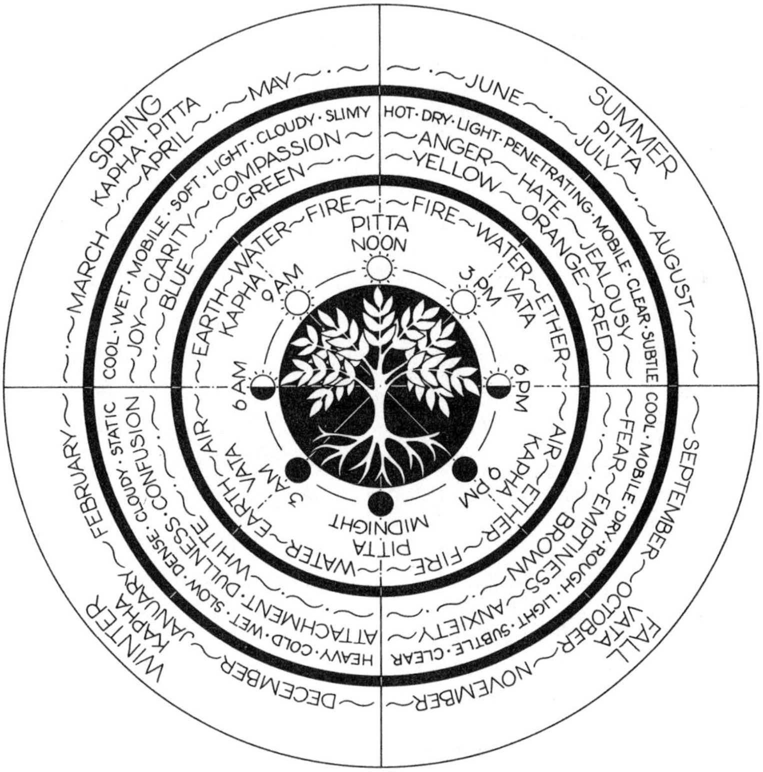

Treatment: tonification and rejuvenation with mainly sweet and pungent herbs to rebuild the body.

PITTA, SAMA: Indications: loss of appetite, little thirst, yellow tongue-coating, urine, feces and mucus yellow or green, heaviness in stomach, thick bilious vomiting, bad breath, bitter or sour taste in mouth, mild burning sensation, skin rash, perception cloudy, conditions may be aggravated by cold.

Treatment: mainly bitter and pungent tasting herbs, bitter tonics and stimulants to clear toxins.

PITTA, NIRAMA: Indications: excessive appetite and thirst, red or inflamed tongue without coating, urine and feces clear, reddish or blackish, strong burning sensations, hot flashes, dizziness, giddiness, perception sharp.

Treatment: cooling and tonifying therapy with mainly sweet and bitter tasting herbs.

KAPHA, SAMA: Indications: mucus cloudy, sticky or thick, does not come out easily, blocks throat, coats tongue, threads form from saliva, sour or salty taste in mouth, congestion, tightness in chest, difficult breathing, mucus in stools and urine, low appetite, heaviness, dull aching, generalized pain, fatigue.

Treatment: mainly pungent and bitter herbs for stimulant and decongestant action to clear toxins, cut mucus and fat.

KAPHA, NIRAMA: Indications: mucus watery, liquid or frothy, comes out easily, sweet taste in mouth, normal appetite, tongue clear, no mucus in stools or urine, no pain.

Treatment: mainly pungent and sweet herbs, expectorants, to clear out excess mucus and *Kapha.*

The usual approach of Ayurveda is to change the *Sama* condition of a *Dosha* to a *Nirama* condition. After the *Ama* is cleared, the *Dosha* can be worked on directly, removing the excesses and tonifying the deficiencies it gives rise to.

HERBAL THERAPEUTICS

ALTERATIVE HERBS (*Rakta Shodhana karma*)

Alteratives are herbs that cleanse and purify the blood. They produce the following general therapeutic effects:

1. They purify the blood, removing toxins, and tend to have anti-infectious, antibacterial action.

2. They help heal and resolve sores, boils, tumors and many kinds of cancer.

3. Typical alteratives work through cooling the blood and so also dispel fevers, reduce *Pitta* and detoxify the liver.

4. They may be used externally on wounds, sores, ulcers, etc. and have anti-inflammatory and vulnerary properties.

5. With their detoxifying action they help kill worms and parasites, particularly those that invade the blood.

6. They work well in infectious, contagious diseases and epidemics.

Alteratives treat flus, especially those with high fever, sore throat, earache, etc.; in this regard they are a degree stronger than cooling diaphoretics. They treat acne, dermatitis, boils and inflammatory skin conditions. They can be used on herpes and venereal diseases, as well as cancer. They cleanse the lymphatics and strengthen white blood cell count. They attack toxic accumulations, but also have a reducing effect upon the bodily tissues. Some possess diuretic or laxative properties.

Most alteratives are cooling, bitter or sometimes astringent in taste. They decrease *Pitta* and *Kapha*, but increase *Vata*. They are mainly anti-*Pitta* herbs.

Typical alteratives (cooling): aloe vera, blue flag, burdock, chaparral, dandelion, echinacea, indigo, *manjishta, neem*, plantain, pokeroot, red clover, sandalwood and yellow dock.

Many hot, pungent herbs possess a cleansing action in the blood, as well as promoting circulation and resolving blood clots. They are detoxifying, often antibacterial, and help reduce fevers by destroying the toxin that produces them. They also have an antiparasitical or worm-killing action.

Hot pungent alteratives and cold bitter alteratives can be combined to strengthen the detoxifying power of each. They can be used together in conditions of high *Ama*. This is true even in *Vata* or *Pitta* constitutions — until the *Ama* is reduced (as in periodic or malarial fevers). Generally speaking, however, cooling alteratives are good for *Pitta*, heating alteratives are good for *Vata*, and both work well on *Kapha*.

Cooling alteratives that have a strong antibacterial or antibiotic effect, like golden seal and wild indigo, if used too long or in excess, can have the same detrimental effect upon the body as antibiotic drugs, destroying the good as well as the bad bacteria in the body, thus weakening the immune system and causing further infections. They must be used with care, particularly when the patient is weak, deficient or emaciated, as in high *Vata* conditions.

Typical heating alteratives include bayberry, blackpepper, cayenne, cinnamon, garlic, myrrh, prickly ash, safflower and sassafras.

Alterative herbs are often taken in the spring as blood-purifiers. This is a good practice, but should not be done in excess, since they may thin the blood, and are not effective in anemic or low blood pressure conditions.

(See also bitter tonic and antipyretic herbs.)

ANTIPARASITICAL AND ANTHELMINTIC HERBS
(*Krumighna karma*)

Anthelmintics are herbs that help destroy and dispel worms. In Ayurveda, the concept of *krumi*, often translated as "worm", has broader implications. It includes all parasites, bacterial, fungal and yeast infections, which were accessible to the subtle vision of the yogis. Anthelmintics are useful in these conditions as well. They have value in treating the widespread yeast infection of Candida albicans, and related food allergy problems.

Parasitical infections are treated like *Ama*, as undigested food while it stagnates will eventually breed some sort of parasite. They are treated with a detoxifying therapy; tonification would only feed the infestation. For this reason anthelmintic herbs have an emaciating effect upon the body and can weaken the tissues. In this regard, sperm is also considered a kind of worm or *krumi*. Anthelmintic herbs may reduce sperm and deplete vitality. Therefore, we should use these herbs symptomatically and with care, especially when the patient is already weak or emaciated.

Ayurveda identifies parasites with the aggravated *Dosha* through which they are manifested. *Kapha*-type parasites reside primarily in mucus or phlegm; *Pitta*-type parasites in the blood; and *Vata*-type parasites are found in the feces. Care must be taken to treat the aggravated *Dosha* as well as the specific parasites.

Antiparasitical action is possessed mainly by pungent or bitter-tasting herbs, yet it is often more a matter of special potency, *Prabhava*, than of general energetics. Still we should be cautious in using hot, pungent anthelmintics on *Pitta*-types or cold, bitter ones on *Vata*-types.

Typical antiparasitical herbs: *ajwan*, asafoetida, cayenne pepper, cloves, garlic, golden seal, pennyroyal, pomegranate, prickly ash, pumpkin seeds, rue, tansy, thyme, wormseed and wormwood.

Worms and parasites often cause an acute condition which should be referred to a qualified practitioner.

ASTRINGENT HERBS (*Stambhana karma*)

Herbs astringent in taste exert a firming, condensing and compacting action upon the tissues and organs of the body. They stop excessive discharges and secretions. Although drying, they are also moisture preserving. In addition, they have a healing action upon skin and mucous membranes.

Astringent taste may be differentiated from astringent action in the following way: astringent tasting herbs have astringent action while herbs of other tastes may also have astringent effects upon the body.

Astringent tasting herbs are mainly used symptomatically, as in stopping bleeding or stopping diarrhea. Yet they often do not correct the condition from which the problem arises. Other herbs of different tastes may, in correcting conditions, alleviate these symptoms also. Diarrhea, for example, may be due to poor absorption in the small intestine. An astringent taste herb like alum or raspberry may suppress the symptom, but will not improve absorption (astringent taste is heavy and difficult to digest). In this regard, an herb like nutmeg, which is pungent and astringent, and which contains heating and digestion promoting action along with astringent action, is more the herb of choice.

It may not always be good to suppress discharges. Diarrhea caused by *Ama* may be the body's way of naturally cleansing itself. To suppress such diarrhea with astringent taste herbs would be to hold the toxins in the body and cause further complications. The correct treatment in this case would be to promote the diarrhea with laxatives until the *Ama* is dispelled. Astringents would only be employed if the diarrhea continued beyond the point of cleansing.

It is important, therefore, that we do not abuse astringent herbs by using them symptomatically like drugs, without understanding the deeper causes of the disorders they may superficially treat.

Ayurveda distinguishes between three different kinds of astringent action: those which stop bleeding, hemostatic herbs (*rakta stambhana*; those which stop excessive discharge of waste materials (*mala stambhana*) and could be called antidiarrhea herbs; and the third group vulnerary herbs (*ropana*), which promote healing of tissues, particularly for external usage. Not all of these herbs are astringent in taste.

Hemostatic herbs stop bleeding, usually by cooling the blood. They are related to alterative herbs, blood-purifiers. Since they are mainly anti-*Pitta* in action, they can aggravate *Vata*. Their taste is usually astringent or bitter.

Typical hemostatic herbs include agrimony, bistort, cattail, golden seal, hibiscus, *manjishta*, marshmallow, mullein, nettle, plantain, red raspberry, saffron, self-heal, shepherd's purse, turmeric, white oak and yarrow.

Some hot pungent herbs have a hemostatic action, particularly where bleeding is caused by cold, as in some *Vata* or *Kapha* conditions. Such herbs include black pepper, cayenne, cinnamon and ginger. These stop bleeding in short term usage but in longer usage may promote bleeding by heating the blood.

Bitter tonics and alterative herbs, which generally cool blood and *Pitta*, may help stop bleeding by their cooling action even without any more specific hemostatic properties.

Astringent action herbs that stop diarrhea may also help eliminate excessive sweating, urination and spontaneous seminal emission. They are usually cooling in energy and astringent to bitter in taste.

Typical antidiarrhea herbs include blackberry, comfrey, cranesbill, gentian, lotus seeds, plantain, red raspberry, sumach, white pond lily, white oak bark and yellow dock.

Some warming herbs also stop diarrhea and other excessive discharges and are usually better for digestion. Such herbs are healthful to *Vata*. They include black pepper, ginger, *haritaki*, nutmeg and poppy seeds. Such substances as buttermilk (*takra*), and yogurt also work on this level.

Vulnerary herbs promote healing of damaged tissue from cuts, wounds, burns, hemorrhaging, etc. They are often used externally in poultices and plasters. Mainly astringent or sweet in taste and cooling in energy, they reduce *Pitta* and *Kapha*. Yet they are not so much for deep-seated injuries where there is much tissue damage, because this requires more tonification (what is usually a more *Vata* condition). Many are demulcent and emollient; softening and soothing to the skin and mucous membranes. Some may contain mucilage.

Typical vulnerary herbs include aloe vera, chickweed, comfrey, honey, marshmallow, plantain, self-heal, shepherd's purse, slippery elm and turmeric.

Some herbs possess all three of these astringent actions and have thereby become famous as heal-all herbs. Such herbs include comfrey, marshmallow, plantain, self-heal and yarrow.

The healing action of astringent herbs is not usually of a nutritive nature. Astringent herbs promote the healing of tissues, but do not actually promote the increase of tissue. This drying action can have not only a healing, but also a wasting effect. Wrong or excessive use of astringent herbs may aggravate *Vata*. This can cause constipation, gas pain, muscle spasms and nervousness.

For this reason, astringent herbs are often used synergistically with nutritive or tonic herbs. The nutritive herbs build up the tissue and the astringents give it firmness and help hold it in the body. Herbs that combine astringent and tonic action are thereby powerful rejuvenatives like *amalaki, bibhitaki* and *haritaki*, three of Ayurveda's most powerful regenerative herbs.

BITTER TONIC AND ANTIPYRETIC HERBS

The Ayurvedic concept of tonic herbs is different than that of most American and European herbal treatments. In western herbalism, the term tonic, which implies an agent that nurtures and strengthens the body, is usually given to cold bitter herbs like gentian or golden seal. These are thought to increase vitality by stimulating digestion. By increasing nutrition the herbs are thought to strengthen the body and its organs, while at the same time giving proper tone to muscles and tissues. This herbal action is said to increase the elimination of toxins, waste-products, and to purify the blood. Tonic herbs are thus prescribed for any convalescent or run-down patient.

In Ayurveda, the use of bitter herbs as tonics is not always appropriate or helpful. Bitter taste, as indicated in our chapter on herbal energetics, is the coldest, most drying, most depletive and reductive of tastes. It is not tonic in the sense of being nutritive—promoting tissue growth or building up the body. Its effects are of a catabolic or reducing nature, detoxifying, promoting the depletion or elimination of tissue, while depressing or sedating most of the organic functions of the body.

Its proper use is more in reducing toxins and excesses, not in building-up deficiencies. Bitter herbs are part of a purification, sedation, heat-dispelling or reducing therapy, which usage they also share in Chinese medicine.

Ayurveda believes that bitter herbs stimulate digestion, but only in small amounts, and mainly for patients suffering from heat, fever or high *Pitta* conditions. They are not often prescribed for the chronically weak or emaciated. Higher dosages are thought to depress digestion, weaken assimilation and derange peristalsis.

Bitter herbs, by their nature as air and ether, dry up the tissues and vital fluids and may cause rigidity of the muscles or even muscle spasms. Rather than promote proper tone of muscles, organs and tissues, under many conditions bitter herbs will reduce it.

While most western herbalism prescribes these herbs for convalescence and debility, Ayurveda often regards them as unhelpful in such conditions. Many cases of weakness and convalescence are *Vata* in nature, conditions of chill, fluid deficiency and the wasting away of bodily tissues. They require a warming, moistening and nutritive therapy. Bitter herbs are also *Vata*, airy in nature, and so provide nothing to rebuild the body or increase vital fluids. It is mainly in conditions of lingering fever, remittent or intermittent, or in the debility following a fever or high *Pitta* state that they can be strengthening.

Perhaps earlier western herbalists used bitter herbs as tonics for convalescence in patients of *Pitta* constitution who suffered from febrile diseases, or had an overdose of toxins from heavy meat-eating, drinking of alcohol and so on. Modern vegetarians, particularly those of *Vata* constitution, would be weakened by over-use of bitter herbs as tonics.

Tonic herbs in Ayurveda are generally sweet, nutritive substances that build tissue, strengthen vitality, increase vital fluids, improve sexual energy and aid longevity. They are considered in a separate section on tonic herbs. Bitter herbs can deplete vitality, depress sexual energy and promote the aging-process. We refer to them in this book as bitter tonics mainly for the sake of convenience, as they are known by this term. We also call them "antipyretics" or herbs which dispel heat, fire and fever.

One could say, with some justification, that these bitter tonics are tonics for *Pitta*, as they are the strongest herbs to reduce and regulate its function. But their action should not be confused with tonics that are nutritive and rejuvenative.

Bitter tonics are, nonetheless, very important herbal medicines. Ayurveda and western herbalism agree that these are the strongest herbs to bring down fevers, to cleanse the body and to kill toxins. They reduce fever, *Pitta*, toxins and fat from the body. They are the strongest herbs for clearing heat.

When the fever is due to an external pathogen and is mainly a surface condition, like the fever due to colds or flus, it should be treated with a diaphoretic therapy by inducing sweating to open the pores, restore circulation and dispel the chill causing it. However, when the fever is high, in the blood or the interior of the body, heating the liver, when there is much thirst, sweating, inflammation or infection, usually a *Pitta* condition, then these bitter tonics are more appropriate.

Bitter tonics do not merely suppress the fever. They destroy the infection which causes it, catabolizing the pathogen. They attack and destroy the *Ama*, the toxins which have entered into the tissues and caused the fever. They are thus indicated in any fever due to *Ama* (which, as in arthritis, may be owing to aggravation of *Vata* or *Kapha*). By their light nature they destroy *Ama*, which is heavy.

In reducing heat, acidity and toxicity, they cool and detoxify the blood; they also possess an alterative or blood-purifying action. One could say that they are like alteratives, but are a degree stronger in action.

They regulate liver function, and control and reduce the production of bile and acid in the body. As such, they are indicated in most liver diseases like hepatitis and jaundice, particularly in the initial and acute phases.

They reduce fat and regulate sugar metabolism. In this way they also regulate spleen functioning and may be helpful in such conditions as diabetes. As the strongest herbs to dispel fat and reduce weight, they have a strong anti-*Kapha* action.

This, along with their blood-purifying action, gives them anti-tumor properties. They may help reduce both benign and malignant tumors, as in cancer. As they catalyze the catabolic processes of the body, they scrape away heavy accretions and remove congestion in the body.

While being the strongest herbs to decrease *Pitta*, and while having a strong reducing action on *Kapha* as well, they are also the strongest herbs to aggravate *Vata*. If we use them in *Vata*-caused indigestion (nervous indigestion, which may be thought to be hypoglycemia) they may only induce further nervous derangements and more hypersensitivity.

Their strong destructive powers may give them antibacterial, antiviral, anthelmintic and antiparasitical properties. Care should be taken to use them only to the point when these pathogens are destroyed; beyond that their destructive powers will weaken the body's own tissues.

Typical bitter tonic and antipyretic herbs include aloe vera, American colombo, barberry, calumba, chaparral, gentian, golden seal, gold thread, Peruvian bark, white poplar, and, special to India, *chirata, kutki* and *neem*.

CARMINATIVE HERBS (*Vata-anuloman*)

Carminatives are herbs that relieve intestinal gas, pain and distention. They settle digestion and increase absorption. They help dispel water and mucus, *Ama*, stagnating in and clogging the gastrointestinal (g.i.) tract. They promote proper and normal peristalsis.

They are usually aromatic or fragrant herbs that possess a volatile oil that stimulates the gastrointestinal nerves (*samana* and *apana vayus*, the forces of *Vata* that govern the stomach, small intestine and colon) to promote digestion and dispel accumulation of undigested food materials.

Their stimulation of *Vata* also increases *Agni*—just as wind increases fire. In this regard, they resemble stimulant herbs as well as other herbs possessing actions in both these categories. But while stimulant herbs tend to promote digestion through a direct feeding of *Agni*, these work more indirectly through normalizing *Vata*. As such they are particularly good for digestive weakness owing to nervous upset, anxiety and depression.

They are closely related to nervines. By dissolving blockages in all the channels, *srotas*, they open up the nervous system and relieve spasms and pain. They may also possess diaphoretic and expectorant action, and are often circulatory stimulants. They improve the general spirit and promote the basic energy flow, *prana*, of the body.

All carminative herbs move *Vata*. This stimulating action moves out accumulated *Vata*. Yet their dryness may aggravate *Vata*, if used too long or in excess.

Most of these aromatic herbs tend to be heating and are usually pungent in taste. A secondary group, however, is cooling and tends towards bitter taste.

Heating carminatives may aggravate *Pitta* and some promote acidity, in which case cooling carminatives would be preferred. Cooling carminatives are more likely to have a long term depleting effect on *Vata*. All aromatic and carminative herbs reduce *Kapha*, owing to their drying property.

Most spices are in this category of herbs, and used as spices they should be part of the daily diet, particularly for someone with a *Vata* constitution. One to five grams of many of these spices taken with meals can cure many diseases, as most disease arises from indigestion. With food or tonic herbs these spices aid in rejuvenation. They correct many congestive diseases and nervous disorders.

Typical heating carminatives: *ajwan*, asafoetida, basil, bay leaves, calamus, cardamom, cinnamon, cloves, garlic, ginger, juniper berries, nutmeg, orange peel, oregano, thyme, turmeric, valerian.

Typical cooling carminatives: chamomile, catnip, chrysanthemum, coriander, cumin, dill, fennel, lime, musta, peppermint, spearmint, wintergreen. (See also stimulant and digestive herbs.)

DIAPHORETIC HERBS (*Svedana karma*)

Diaphoretic herbs induce perspiration and by this action restore circulation, dispel fever and chills, while eliminating toxins from the surface of the body. Strong diaphoretics are called sudorifics.

They are surface-relieving agents used in the initial and acute stages of colds and flus, as well as more chronic conditions of asthma and arthritis. The initial or acute stage of colds and febrile diseases paralyzes the defensive energy that moves along the surface of the body. The result is a stoppage of sweating and a blockage of circulation. Diaphoretic herbs, by stimulating, restore the defensive energy of the body.

They produce the following general therapeutic effects: a) promote sweating, b) relieve muscle tension and aching joints, c) bring down fevers due to external factors (associated with colds and flus), d) promote the eruption and resolution of inflammatory skin conditions, e) help disperse surface water and facial edema and f) relieve headaches due to cold and congestion. As such they are the first line of defense against disease.

Ayurveda recognizes two kinds of diaphoretic herbs according to the *Dosha* on which they work. These two kinds are warming and cooling diaphoretics.

Most diaphoretics are of the warming nature. They are generally hot, pungent herbs that decrease *Kapha* and *Vata* but increase *Pitta*. Most colds are of a *Kapha* nature, an invasion of chill and damp. *Vata*, or wind, is the factor that carries them into the body. Warming diaphoretics treat the common cold by dispersing wind, chill and dampness. They are generally stimulants, expectorants and may possess antiasthmatic and antirheumatic properties.

Cooling diaphoretics are usually bitter-to-pungent herbs that decrease *Pitta* and *Kapha* but increase *Vata*. They are more for *Pitta*-type colds and are more effective in treating high fever, sore throat and other inflammatory symptoms involving the invasion of toxins in the blood. They are generally alteratives and may possess diuretic properties.

Warming diaphoretics raise body temperature and through sweating, they dispel chills. Cooling diaphoretics lower body temperature through sweating, and dispel heat and toxins through the skin. Both dispel water, phlegm and *Kapha*.

Kapha-constitution requires strong diaphoresis owing to its wet attribute. *Pitta*-constitution requires moderate diaphoresis of a cooling nature. It can be aggravated by heating diaphoretics, by hot sweat or steam baths, or by hot tubs and saunas, which relieve *Kapha*. *Vata* requires mild diaphoresis of a predominately warming nature to help moisten its surface dryness, but strong diaphoretic methods may dry *Vata* out further.

It should be remembered that colds and flus (as initial and surface diseases) may not be of the same *Dosha* as the constitution of the person. A *Pitta* person may have a *Kapha* cold—most colds are *Kapha*, at least in the beginning. For such temporary diseases, our treatment can be symptomatic.

Diaphoretics cleanse the lymphatics and the plasma, Ayurvedic *Rasa Dhatu*. Cooling diaphoretics may also have a cleansing action of the blood. Diaphoretics help cleanse the subtle channels and capillaries. They work primarily on the lungs and the respiratory system. Yet they also help open the mind and breath, increase *Prana*, clear the sinuses and the senses and stimulate the nervous system. Cooling diaphoretics have additional cleansing action on the liver and blood.

In Ayurveda diaphoresis is part of the preliminary treatment in *Pancha Karma*, or purification therapy. After oil massage, which softens the toxins in the body, it is used to melt them and render them mobile for elimination from the body. Diaphoresis usually is followed by emesis, purgation or enema as prime therapy, but it may sometimes be a prime therapy in itself.

Diaphoresis does not require herbs but can be done through fire, steam, exercise, hot baths and so on. The use of herbal diaphoretics should be included with a hot bath, sleeping under a warm blanket and fasting.

Typical heating diaphoretics: angelica, basil, bayberry, camphor, cardamom, cinnamon, cloves, ephedra (ma huang), eucalyptus, ginger, juniper berries, sage, thyme, wild ginger.

Typical cooling diaphoretics: boneset, burdock, catnip, chamomile, chrysanthemum, coriander, elder flowers, horehound, horsetail, peppermint, spearmint, yarrow.

DIURETIC HERBS (*Mutrala karma*)

Diuretic herbs increase urination. They promote the functional

activity of the kidneys and urinary bladder. Acting on the water element
in all the tissue-elements (*dhatus*) of the body, diuretic herbs reduce and
remove toxins.

Their action is largely one of detoxification and purgation through the
urine. They are purgatives for the water element in the body and as such
they reduce the earth element in the body. Hence, like all purgatives, they
must be used with caution.

Diuretics decrease water and reduce *Kapha*, whose main constituent
is water. Generally they are bitter, astringent or pungent in taste. Similarly,
all diuretics tend to increase the dryness of *Vata*. This action is aggravated
by the tastes that relieve *Kapha* and dampness.

Diuretics also reduce *Pitta*. Many or even most of them are stronger
in reducing *Pitta* than *Kapha*. This is not just because *Pitta* is also somewhat oily in nature. It is because urination is also a way of relieving heat
from the body; of removing acid and toxins from the blood; a way of
cooling and purifying the blood. This relieves *Pitta*.

Heating and drying herbs, pungent taste, bring water up and out of
the body through the process of sweating—diaphoretic action. They also
work by relieving mucus through the mouth in expectoration. Just as
water evaporates upwards by the action of fire, heating and drying herbs
purify our system.

Cooling and drying herbs, bitter and astringent tastes—on the other
hand—bring water downwards through the urine. Cold herbs cause a
descending or contracting action, the way hot herbs create a rising and
dispersing action.

Diuretic action is generally cooling and drying—the opposite of the
qualities of *Pitta*, heat and moisture. For this reason, diuretics dispel damp
heat, as in diarrhea and dysentery, and cool down not only the kidneys
and bladder, but also the liver and gall bladder. In increasing urination,
they help dispel kidney and bladder stones, and also stones of the gall
bladder. Such stone-dispelling herbs are called lithotriptic.

In their more specific anti-*Kapha* action, diuretic herbs dispel edema
and water accumulation in the tissues, particularly in the lower half of the
body. (Facially-accumulated water and water in the head and chest are
often better reduced by diaphoretic and expectorant herbs.) They help
decrease fat and reduce weight, particularly when fat is mainly composed
of water.

They stimulate bladder and kidney function, but are seldom actually tonic or nutritive to the kidneys. Their drying action may cause constipation or dryness of the skin. Scanty urination without water accumulation requires a moistening, not a drying therapy, and in that condition, diuretic herbs are usually contraindicated. Vata constitution needs to increase urine by increasing water in the tissues—not a diuretic but a tonic or nutritive therapy. Diuretics are probably the strongest herbs to aggravate Vata, and are contraindicated in conditions of convalescent debility and dehydration.

Diuretics can be divided into cooling and heating kinds, the cooling types are in the majority. Cooling diuretics are often also cooling diaphoretics, alteratives or antipyretic herbs, useful in fevers and infectious diseases, particularly those involving the urino-genital tract (as herpes) or the liver and gall bladder.

Warming diuretics, like juniper berries, are often warming diaphoretics, stimulants and expectorants and may have antirheumatic action. They are contraindicated in Pitta conditions of kidney or gall bladder inflammation unless they are balanced out by a majority of cooling herbs.

A few diuretics are cooling and moistening, apart from their drying action in diuresis, and have a soothing effect upon the mucous membranes of the urinary system. Examples are marshmallow, barley or gokshura. Often one such herb is added to a diuretic formula to soothe and protect the kidneys from the drying and scraping action of diuretic herbs that can cause irritation and discomfort.

Typical cooling diuretics: asparagus, barley, buchu, burdock, cleavers, coriander, cornsilk, dandelion, fennel, gokshura, gravel root, horsetail, lemon grass, marshmallow, plantain, punarnava, spearmint, uva ursi.

Typical warming diuretics: ajwan, cinnamon, cubebs, garlic, juniper berries, Mormon tea, mustard, parsley, wild carrot.

EMMENAGOGUES (Raktabhisarana karma)

Emmenagogues are herbs that help promote and regulate menstruation and thereby treat many of the special disorders of the female reproductive system; these include P.M.S., uterine tumors or infections. Such herbs are called raktabhisarana, herbs that promote the flow of blood, in Ayurveda, what could be called "circulatory stimulants."

Emmenagogues are largely pungent-to-bitter herbs that relieve congestion of the blood, clear blood clots and promote menstruation. They warm the blood and improve its quality, stimulating the heart. They may be heating or cooling in energy, with those cooling in the majority.

The female reproductive system is intimately associated with the blood; it is, therefore, *Pitta* in nature. Imbalances should be examined as increased or decreased *Pitta* conditions. Naturally, the same treatment cannot work in both cases. Those emmenagogues that are cooling in nature are better for high *Pitta* menstrual disorders; those heating in nature for low *Pitta*.

A predominance of cooling emmenagogues is better for menstrual irregularities owing to such conditions as uterine infection or bleeding. Such herbs also help calm high emotions, anger and irritability. A predominance of heating emmenagogues is better for delayed menstruation due to exposure to cold, overexertion or nervous anxiety.

Emmenagogues may also be antispasmodics, relieving uterine cramping and pain. Those which are diuretic treat pre-menstrual water retention. Those which are hemostatic are better for excessive menstruation.

Typical heating emmenagogues: angelica, asafoetida, cinnamon, cotton root, ginger, mugwort, myrrh, parsley, pennyroyal, safflower, tang kuei, turmeric, valerian.

Typical cooling emmenagogues: blessed thistle, chamomile, chrysanthemum, hibiscus, *manjishta*, motherwort, musta, primrose, red raspberry, rose flowers, squawvine, yarrow.

Emmenagogues work largely by increasing *apana vayu*, the downward-moving *Vata* governing elimination, urination and sexual functions. As such, they tend to be laxative and to promote the discharge of the fetus. Hence, many are contraindicated during pregnancy.

Ayurveda distinguishes another group of emmenagogues—those which are tonic or rejuvenative to the female reproductive system. These are a subcategory of tonic, rejuvenative and aphrodisiac herbs. They are mainly sweet herbs that build the blood, moisten and nourish the female reproductive organs, and so treat conditions of organ weakness due to disease, poor nutrition or the effects of aging.

Typical tonic and rejuvenative emmenagogues: aloe vera, angelica, cotton root, false unicorn, licorice, lotus seeds, myrrh, peony, *rehmannia*, *shatavari*, Solomon's seal, wild yam, and such flowers as hibiscus, jasmine, rose and saffron. In this regard, Ayurveda also uses various iron preparations.

EXPECTORANT AND DEMULCENT HERBS
(Kasa-Svasahara)

Expectorant herbs promote the discharge of phlegm and mucus from the body. They clear the lungs and nasal passages, but also the stomach. They are useful in respiratory afflictions, chronic or acute colds, flus, asthma, bronchitis, pneumonia. Such problems Ayurveda refers to as *kasa* and *svasa*, which mean literally cough and dyspnea (difficult breathing).

They may also be helpful in digestive problems because mucus has its origin in the stomach and may clog the gastrointestinal tract, giving rise to indigestion and poor assimilation.

Phlegm and mucus can accumulate anywhere in the body, causing various growths or tumors (generally benign). They may accumulate under the skin, for example, and can clog the channels of the circulatory and other systems, leading to all manner of diseases, including nervous disorders.

Expectorant herbs are of two kinds and work in two different ways. Some expectorants, like ginger, remove mucus by a drying action. They are mainly pungent in taste and hot in energy, and may also be stimulant, diaphoretic or carminative herbs. (A few, however, like horehound, are bitter in taste and cooling in energy and are particularly good for *Pitta*.)

Others, like licorice, help remove mucus by a moistening action. They increase and liquify *Kapha*, promoting its flow out of the body. They are mainly sweet and cold herbs. These are also demulcent and emollient herbs, mucilaginous substances that have a softening and soothing effect upon the skin and mucous membranes.

Warming and drying expectorants dispel chill and dampness, decrease *Kapha* and *Ama*, increase *Pitta* and *Agni*, and are particularly good for *Kapha* or *Kapha-Vata* type colds and respiratory afflictions.

Cooling and moistening expectorants dispel heat and dryness, liquify *Kapha* and *Ama*, and work more on *Vata* or *Pitta-Vata* type colds and respiratory, afflictions of sore throat or dry, hacking cough.

Most expectorants possess cough-relieving action, as coughs are usually caused by mucus blockage or irritation of the respiratory passages. Hence we include most cough-relieving herbs in this category (though some possess more specific action from nervine or antispasmodic properties).

Coughs should similarly be discriminated as wet (productive) or dry (unproductive) and treated with the appropriate kinds of herbs. Cough or cold with clear, abundant phlegm usually indicates *Kapha* disorder, chill-damp. Cough or cold with yellow phlegm or inflammation of the mucous membranes usually indicates fever or *Pitta* derangement, damp-heat. Dry cough along with scanty phlegm and chill usually indicates *Vata*, particularly if it is a chronic condition.

Coughs and colds are basically *Kapha* disorders, as mucus is *Kapha* and *Kapha* has as its site the stomach and lungs. Chronic colds and mucous congestion are often relieved by therapeutic vomiting, emetic therapy, a kind of radical expectorant action.

Moistening expectorants or demulcents can be used externally to help heal sores, wounds or ulcers. They are nutritive and promote cell growth, as well as being anti-inflammatory.

They are the closest category in western herbology to true tonics in the Ayurvedic sense; sweet, nutritive herbs that directly feed and strengthen the organs and tissues. They can be called lung tonics. Some have rejuvenative action. By their softening action, some are laxatives.

The soothing action of demulcent herbs gives them a power to help calm the heart and nerves. They are effective nervines in *Vata* conditions of dehydration and tissue depletion. Demulcent herbs alleviate dryness-caused friction that irritates physiological function. They feed the mucous membranes and the connective tissue.

Both kinds of expectorants may be combined to help balance their action. Hot, dry expectorants, like ginger, may be used with a moistening expectorant like licorice, so as not to aggravate *Vata* or *Pitta* by its dryness or heat. Cold, moist expectorants may require the addition of a hot, pungent herb like ginger, as they are heavy and hard to digest and may aggravate *Ama*. The effect of a formula depends upon the predomination of herbs in it and should not be too one-sided in action.

Typical drying expectorants: boneset, calamus, cardamom, cinnamon, cloves, cubebs, elecampane, ginger (dry), horehound, hyssop, mustard seeds, orange peel, *pippali*, sage, wild ginger, yerba santa.

Typical moistening expectorants or demulcents: bamboo (*vamsha rochana*), chickweed, comfrey root, flaxseed, Irish moss, licorice, maidenhair fern, marshmallow, milk, raw sugar, slippery elm, Solomon's seal.

Typical cough-relieving herbs: apricot seeds, bayberry, coltsfoot, ephedra (ma huang), eucalyptus, grindelia, horehound, mullein, osha, thyme, wild cherry.

LAXATIVE AND PURGATIVE HERBS (*Virechana karma*)

Laxative herbs promote bowel movements, dispel constipation, and help eliminate food accumulations and toxic build-ups from the intestines. They may be weak or strong. Weak laxatives are called simply laxatives or aperients. Strong laxatives are called purgatives or cathartics.

Purgatives promote forceful evacuation, and may cause diarrhea and griping, with perhaps pain and tenesmus, owing to what is often an irritant effect. As such, they should be used with care. Purgatives are usually either cold, bitter herbs like rhubarb or hot oils like castor oil.

Mild laxatives are mainly moistening herbs and bulk laxatives, like bran. They work through increasing elimination through greater lubrication of the intestines. Some cold, bitter herbs, like cascara sagrada, also have a mild laxative action, but it is more like a weak purgative, working through stimulating peristalsis.

Laxatives and purgatives are indicated wherever there is constipation, or wherever there is a pronounced coating at the back of the tongue, denoting a build-up of toxins in the colon. Sometimes a person who has regular bowel movements may still have a large accumulation of fecal matter in the colon and so require purgation. Whenever there are toxins in the colon, which may also cause diarrhea, purgatives can be used. They can also be used in the later stages of a fever to help clear the toxins out of the body.

Chronic constipation, as well as constipation in the elderly, is usually a *Vata* condition, with its accumulation of gas and dryness in the colon. For this condition, generally mild, moistening or bulk laxatives are prescribed; strong purgatives would cause irritation. However, sometimes a strong purge is necessary for high build-up of toxins due to accumulated *Vata*. In such cases, the hot oils, like castor, are specific.

Pitta constitution tends towards diarrhea due to its damp attribute, but where heat is high it may also cause constipation. Either way, purgatives of a usually cold and bitter nature, which work on the small intestine, are prescribed. Purgation (*virechana*) is the strongest way to eliminate *Pitta*, heat and bile from the body.

However, where there is inflammation or ulceraton of the intestinal membranes, which is usually a *Pitta* condition, strong purgatives can cause irritation. For such condition moistening laxatives of a cooling nature, like psyllium seeds, would be indicated.

Kapha constitution may be constipated owing to the accumulation of phlegm, mucus and undigested food particles in the intestines due to deficient digestive power. For this condition, laxatives of a drying nature are indicated; bulk or moistening laxatives would increase congestion.

Laxatives tend to suppress the power of digestion, and may weaken peristalsis in the long run by over stimulation. As such they should be used with stimulant or carminative herbs, like ginger and fennel seeds. Constipation or toxins in the colon can also be treated by increasing the power of digestion, *Agni*. Hot, spicy stimulant-carminative herbs can help correct constipation in a *Vata* or *Kapha* constitution without actually having to use laxatives. Dryness in the colon may also be related to dryness in the lungs, and herbs that moisturize the lungs also, like licorice or flaxseed, may be more specific to the condition.

Typical moistening or bulk laxatives: bran, flaxseed, ghee, licorice, prunes, psyllium seed, raisins, *shatavari*, warm milk.

Strong purgatives: aloe vera (powder), castor oil, croton, epsom salt, mandrake, rhubarb, senna.

Cooling herbs with various degrees of laxative action: aloe vera, blue flag, cascara sagrada, echinacea, gentian, rhubarb, senna, yellow dock.

Strong purgatives and mild laxatives may be combined for moderate action; the divisions, again, are not rigid.

NERVINE AND ANTISPASMODIC HERBS

Nervines are herbs that strengthen the functional activity of the nervous system. They may be stimulants or sedatives and can be used to correct excesses or deficiencies of nervous function. They have a strong action on the mind and are useful in promoting mental health and clarity as well as aiding in the treatment of psychological imbalances and mental diseases.

Most nervines are also antispasmodics; herbs that relieve spasms of the voluntary or involuntary muscles and thereby relieve cramps, stop tremors and convulsions. They may also serve as broncho-dilators, stopping spasms in the bronchial tubes, thus proving effective for respiratory afflictions. Others may help relieve menstrual cramping and headaches.

Many of these herbs are fragrant, aromatic herbs like mint or valerian. This is because aromatic herbs work directly on *Prana*, the prime energy of the nervous system, as they are themselves substances that contain much *Prana* (the air element). Such aromatic herbs open the mind and senses, clear the channels (*srotas*), relieve congestion, stop pain and restore the smooth flow of energy in the body-mind system.

Aromatic nervines are often also carminative and stomachic herbs, herbs that dispel intestinal gas and cramping. The basis for this can be seen in light of Ayurvedic physiology. *Vata*, the *Dosha* that governs the nervous system, accumulates in the colon, from which it invades the tissue-elements of the body. It is also in the colon that the assimilation of nutrients, mainly oils, occurs for the sustenance of nerve and bone tissue. Hence the treatment of *Vata* in the colon is often a root treatment for *Vata* in the nervous system; *Vata*-relieving herbs can treat both.

Generally speaking, in Ayurveda we think of nervousness as *Vata* or as the mark of a *Vata* constitution, for *Vata* governs nerve responses and, by nature as air or wind, it is impulsive, vaccillatory, hypersensitive. Most diseases of the nervous system are diseases of *Vata*. Hence, in treating nervous disorders, we must first consider *Vata*. Most nerve pain, lumbago, sciatica, paralysis and degenerative nervous disorders are *Vata* diseases.

Yet many emotional or nervous disorders may be caused by the other *Doshas*, as those due to anger which would be a *Pitta* condition. Or *Vata* may be blocked or aggravated by the other *Doshas*, in which case an apparant *Vata* disorder would be due to an underlying excess of *Pitta* or *Kapha*. So, again, we must locate primary causes rather than evident effects.

Vata-emotions, like fear and anxiety, weaken the kidneys and adrenals. They damage the nerves and cause insomnia, mental instability, nerve pain, cramping and numbness, which may lead eventually to the wasting away of nerve tissue. Most nervines, particularly those which are aromatic, move *Vata* , and so help remove the obstructed *Vata* or life-energy behind these disorders.

A few herbs are not only aromatic, but possess *tamasic*, heavy or dulling properties. These are particularly good for both moving and grounding *Vata*, which suffers from "ungroundedness"—from an excess of air and ether. Such herbs include asafoetida, garlic and valerian.

Yet where there is a deficiency of nerve tissues, often due to poor nutrition, nutritive herbs are needed—*ashwagandha* or licorice (see tonics). Excessive use of aromatic nervines may further weaken the nerves by their drying action; they may also be over-stimulating.

Pitta-type emotions, anger, envy, hatred and so on, heat up the blood, the liver and the heart, creating internal fire. Thereby they can cause hypertension, insomnia, irritability and other mental and nervous imbalances. They can also burn out the nerves, a condition of the high-*Pitta*, aggressive, "business executive's" life style.

Pitta-caused nervous disorders can often be treated with general anti-*Pitta* herbs (see management of *Pitta*) like bitter tonics or purgatives, without having to resort to any specific nervine herbs at all.

Yet many, perhaps most, of the herbs that act upon the mind are cooling in energy. This is because the mind is unbalanced largely by negative emotions, which are like *Pitta* and create heat. A calm and clear mind is usually a cool mind. Hence many herbs for the mind, like gotu kola, are good anti-*Pitta* herbs.

Kapha nervous conditions are more a matter of dullness, lethargy, hypoactivity of the nervous system. Psychologically, *Kapha* suffers from greed, desire, attachment, clinging to the past. In terms of the mind and nerves, *Kapha* requires stimulation. Nervines that are aromatic, stimulant and decongestant are best for *Kapha*, and most aromatics, by their drying nature, are good for *Kapha*.

Herbs that put *Vata* or *Pitta* to sleep may keep *Kapha* awake—skullcap, for example. Herbs affect different *Doshas* differently. What sedates one *Dosha* may stimulate another.

Many herbs that calm the mind tend to have a positive effect on all three *Doshas*, as it is in the balance of the *Doshas* that the mind is calm. Hence, some nervines may be good for all three *Doshas* (*tridosha* herbs), particularly in small amounts or short term usage. Such cooling aromatics as mint, chamomile or fennel can be widely used as mild nervines. Their drying nature relieves *Kapha*; their cooling energy relieves *Pitta*; and their aromatic property removes obstructed *Vata*.

Like other herbal categories, nervines can be divided into heating and cooling types. Cooling nervines are generally better for *Pitta*, heating for *Vata* and *Kapha* (though both kinds reduce *Kapha* and move obstructed

Vata to some degree).

Typical heating nervine and antispasmodic herbs: asafoetida, basil, bayberry, calamus, camphor, eucalyptus, garlic, *guggul*, lady's slipper, mugwort, myrrh, nutmeg, pennyroyal, poppy seeds, sage, valerian.

Typical cooling nervine and antispasmodic herbs: betony, *bhringaraj*, catnip, chamomile, gotu kola, hops, jasmine, *jatamamsi*, motherwort, mullein, oatstraw, passion flower, peppermint, sandalwood, skullcap, spearmint, St. John's Wort, vervain, wild yam.

There are other special nervine herbs that are more like drugs and from which many drugs have been derived. They contain certain chemicals or alkaloids on which their action depends. Such special effects of minute chemicals that transcend the energetics of taste are regarded as examples of *Prabhava*. Their action is strong and their side effects cause paralysis. Most are poisons, severely aggravate *Pitta*, and should be used with care. They are outside the scope of this book, but some are used traditionally in Ayurveda for these special effects. Examples include dhatura (jimsonweed), digitalis, marijuana, opium.

Metals, minerals and gems have special action on the mind and nervous system. Ayurveda includes within its scope special preparations of these, made non-toxic to the human body. Such compounds relate back to the old alchemical tradition and are called *Siddha Yoga* compounds. Many are traceable to the great Buddhist sage *Nagarjuna*, who was also a great Ayurvedic doctor, said to have lived for many centuries. These compounds also relate to longevity therapy (see rejuvenatives, under tonics) and are another special feature of Ayurveda.

STIMULANT AND DIGESTIVE HERBS
(*Dipana-Pachana karma*)

In western herbalism, stimulants are herbs that generally stimulate, increase or promote all organic functions. They do this primarily by stimulating the power of digestion.

Stimulants are mainly hot in energy, pungent in taste, and include most hot spices, peppers and gingers. Their action is to increase internal heat, dispel internal chill, and strengthen the metabolism and circulation.

They are the most powerful herbs to increase *Agni*, the digestive fire, and are thereby the strongest herbs to destroy *Ama*, toxic accumulations. They are synonymous with *Agni Dipana* and *Ama Pachana* herbs in

Ayurveda; herbs that increase *Agni* and digest *Ama*. They contain large amounts of *Agni*, so that even if the body's *Agni* is low, they can still burn away toxins.

They warm the stomach, increase the appetite, warm the blood, and stimulate the senses. They often have antibacterial or antiparasitical powers and increase the auto-immune system. They do not actually build up the body, but they allow for the assimilation of food whereby the body can be built up. They are often used with tonic and nutritive herbs as well as with foods.

They are the most powerful herbs to increase *Pitta* and decrease *Kapha*. Generally, they decrease *Vata*, but in excess they can aggravate it through their drying property.

They are good for *Sama* conditions and can be used in small amounts on *Sama Pitta*. Destroying toxins, they also help relieve fevers, and for this purpose may be combined with bitter tonics and antipyretic herbs.

Many stimulant-digestive herbs have carminative and stomachic properties, as they also stimulate peristalsis (*samana vayu*). Many have diaphoretic properties by heating the surface of the body and promoting sweating. They also increase appetite. Many have expectorant qualities. They help dispel *Kapha* or mucus from the stomach, lungs and nasal passages, and promote the flow of tears. In promoting circulation, they possess some blood-purifying effects.

These digestive stimulants are related to nerve stimulants. They may increase hypertension or cause insomnia. They should be used only to supplement functional weaknesses, not to enable the user to sustain the abuses of excessive activity.

Stimulant and digestive herbs are indicated whenever the digestion is to be improved, cold is to be dispelled, toxins and tongue-coating are to be cleared up, and degenerated metabolism and circulation are to be revived.

They are contraindicated in conditions of dehydration, fluid insufficiency, and inflammatory conditions of the mucous membranes. They should not be directly applied to the mucous membranes.

Typical stimulant herbs: *ajwan*, asafoetida, black pepper, cayenne, cinnamon, cloves, garlic, ginger (dry), horseradish, mustard, onions, *pippali*, prickly ash.

Western herbalism regards some cold bitter herbs or bitter tonics as possessing stimulant action. This is like a cold shower or a quick dip in cold water that serves to warm the body. Ayurveda considers such herbs as better for promoting digestion of toxins than for promoting normal food digestion.

(For such cold, bitter stimulants, see bitter tonic and antipyretic herbs.)

TONICS

A) Nutritive Tonics (*Bruhana karma*)

The Ayurvedic concept of a tonic is a substance that nurtures the tissue-elements (*dhatus*) of the body. A nutritive tonic is an herb that nourishes the body and increases weight, density and substance within it. Such herbal foods serve the various *dhatus* or organs that have been depleted or weakened by disease.

Tonics are usually sweet in taste, or in post-digestive effect, which indicates their constructive action. Generally, they have the same nature as *Kapha* and are composed primarily of earth and water.

Tonics are usually heavy, oily or mucilaginous. They increase vital fluids, muscle and fat and build the blood and lymph, increasing milk and semen. They are restoratives for conditions of weakness, emaciation, debility and convalescence. They have a softening, soothing, harmonizing effect, which dispels rigidity and calms the nerves.

Nutritive tonics generally decrease *Vata* and *Pitta* and increase *Kapha*. A few which are heating, like ginseng or sesame seeds, may aggravate *Pitta*. They increase *Ama* and are not the herbs of choice for *Sama* conditions, though they can help soften *Ama* where other more primary herbs facilitate its discharge. Nutritive tonics are moistening and cooling in energy—the best herbs to reduce the dryness of *Vata*.

Yet they are also heavy and are hard to digest. For the low *Agni*, particularly of *Vata* constitutions, they are usually combined with various stimulant or carminative herbs (e.g. ginger or cardamom) to aid in their absorption.

For *Pitta* conditions, herbs that combine astringent or bitter with sweet taste, like comfrey root or *shatavari*, are most appropriate. With their cooling energy, they can be used in convalescence from high fever, toxic blood, ulcers or other inflammatory *Pitta* conditions.

Many of these nutritive tonic herbs possess expectorant, demulcent and emollient action. They soothe and nurture the mucous membranes and restore bodily fluids and secretions. As such, they are particularly nurturing for the mucous membranes of the lungs and stomach. They have a healing action on the skin and may help soften and relieve muscle tension and pain.

Ayurveda enhances the nutritive action of herbs with other sweet and nutritive substances like milk, *ghee* and raw sugar.

Typical nutritive tonics: almonds, *amalaki*, angelica (tang kuei), *bala*, coconut, comfrey root, dates, flaxseeds, ginseng, honey, Irish moss, licorice, lotus seeds, marshmallow, milk, raisins, rehmannia, saw palmetto, sesame seeds, *shatavari*, slippery elm, Solomon's seal, spikenard, sugar, *vidari kanda*, wild yam.

B) Rejuvenative Tonics (*Rasayana karma*)

Ayurvedic herbology reaches its culmination in the science of rejuvenation. Aimed at renewal of both body and mind, Ayurvedic herbology does not seek simply longevity, but moves towards a life of pure awareness, natural creativity, spontaneous delight.

The approach is not only towards physical immortality (which on some deeper level of harmony may be possible), but the immortality of the mind, the daily renewal of brain cells. In such a state, the mind and heart are as clear in old age as in childhood.

This science is called *Rasayana*. *Rasayana* is what enters (*ayana*), in the essence (*rasa*). It is what penetrates and revitalizes the essence of our psycho-physiological being.

Rasayana substances rebuild the body-mind, prevent decay, and postpone aging. They may even help reverse the aging process. They do not simply add to the bulk or quantity of the body, but increase its quality. *Rasayana* substances are more subtle, more specific, and more lasting than simple nutritive tonics. Their action sustains the optimal form and function of the various organs, *dhatus* and *doshas* in the body. They are not necessarily sweet and nutritive, though most are sweet at least in *vipaka* (post-digestive effect). Rejuvenative tonics for *Kapha* may be pungent and hot.

Rasayana substances often have unique potencies. Their action is determined as much by *prabhava* as by the regular rules of taste and energy.

According to Ayurveda, plants possess *Soma*, which is the ambrosia or nectar of immortality. It is also the subtle invigorating fluid, *Ojas*, the innermost sap of the body. *Soma* (*Ojas*) is the basis for clarity of perception, physical strength, endurance, and longevity of the tissues.

Soma is the subtle essence-energy of the nervous system, the digested essence of all food, impressions and experiences. As such it is our capacity to enjoy life. It was called "the food of the gods," as in it is the capacity to find delight in all things.

The ancient Vedic Science of *Rasayana* was aimed primarily at the mutation of the brain. It attempted to give a physical basis, the right receptacle, for the birth of true awareness in human beings. By transcending the conditioned functioning of the "old brain," with its regressive patterns of fear, desire and ambition based on egoistic function, *Rasayana* performed "miraculous" changes.

The real *Soma* is the purified essence of feeling and sensitivity. Such clarity of awareness is the nectar that feeds and brings about mutation in brain cells.

Today, we no longer know which plant was used as the original *Soma*, if indeed it was the product of a particular plant. However, all *Rasayana* herbs have a similar usage and capacity.

Rasayana treatment includes special herbs, but goes far beyond the bounds of any ordinary medical treatment. It includes *mantra* and meditation, which are the real catalysts for this process.

This highest *Rasayana* treatment of inner transmutation is called *Brahma Rasayana*. *Brahma* (usually called Brahman in English usage) means expansion, and refers to the unbounded expansion that is the creative reality of life. Through meditation, we transcend the limitation of the known, the conditioned functioning of the brain.

Typical *Rasayanas*:

For *Vata*: ashwagandha, calamus, garlic, ginseng, *guggul, haritaki*.
For *Pitta*: aloe vera, *amalaki*, comfrey root, gotu kola, saffron, *shatavari*.
For *Kapha*: *bibhitaki*, elecampane, *guggul, pippali*.

Other *Rasayanas*: angelica (tang kuei), *bala*, fo-ti, *gokshura*, licorice, *manjishta*, marshmallow, myrrh, oatstraw, onion, rehmannia, saw palmetto, sesame seeds, Solomon's seal, spikenard, *vamsha rochana, vidari kanda*, wild yam.

Many herbs possess rejuvenative powers, but to lesser degrees. Other western herbs may have strong rejuvenative powers, but this requires further research.

C) Aphrodisiacs (*Vajikarana*)

A third kind of tonic herb, closely allied with *Rasayanas*, is what is called in Ayurveda *Vijakarana*. A *vaji* is a horse or stallion. These are substances that give the power or vitality of a horse, particularly the horse's great capacity for sexual activity. More commonly, one could call them "aphrodisiacs," though they are much more than superstitious love potions. *Vajikaranas* reinvigorate the body by reinvigorating the sexual organs.

The semen or reproductive tissue (the Ayurvedic concept includes both male and female reproductive tissues) is the essence of all the *dhatus*, the cream of all the tissue-elements in the body. It contains the power to create life. This means not only the capacity to bring a new life into existence, to create a child, but also to renew one's own life, to return our cells to the vigor of youth. That same life-creating energy, if directed inwards, can aid in the renewal of both body and mind.

Vajikarana substances may be used either to improve sexual vitality and functioning, or to help direct sexual energy inwards for regeneration. Most of these are not simple aphrodisiacs—substances exciting sexual activity through irritation of the sexual organs. Many are tonics that actually nurture and give direct sustenance to the reproductive tissues. Others help promote the creative transformation of sexual energy for the benefit of the body-mind.

By starting in the reproductive system, these herbs invigorate the entire system, just as a tree is invigorated from the roots. They have a strong revitalizing action on the nerves and bone marrow, and increase the energy of the mind. Semen is the *Soma* of the body, which if catalyzed in the right way, by *Rasayana* and *Vajikarana* substances, brings about the renewal of the mind. In a similar way it helps strengthen the bones, muscles, ligaments and blood.

Vajikaranas can be divided into tonics and stimulants. Stimulants increase the functional activity of the reproductive organs, while tonics increase and improve the tissue-substance that composes them. Many aphrodisiacs increase *Kapha*; some which are hot and pungent increase *Pitta*.

Typical aphrodisiacs (*Vajikaranas*): angelica (tang kuei), asafoetida, *ashwagandha*, asparagus, cloves, cotton root, damiana, false unicorn, fenugreek, fo-ti, garlic, ginseng, *gokshura*, hibiscus, lotus seeds, onions (raw), *pippali*, rehmannia, rose, saffron, saw palmetto, *shatavari*, Solomon's seal, *vidari-kanda*, wild yam. Of these, those which are emmenagogues are more specific for women.

Ayurveda also discriminates those herbs that enhance spermatogenesis, called *Shukrala*. These are substances that are nutritive tonics to the reproductive secretions, like semen and breast milk. They are mainly those *Vajikaranas* which are nutritive.

Such nutritive aphrodisiacs include: angelica (tang kuei), *ashwagandha, bala*, fo-ti, ghee, ginseng, licorice, lotus seeds, marshmallow, onions (raw), rehmannia, saw palmetto, sesame seeds, *shatavari*, Solomon's seal, sugar (raw), *vidari-kanda*, wild yam.

Those aphrodisiacs whose nature is *sattvic*, and are strong in energy, also enhance *Ojas*. Such substances include *ashwagandha, ghee*, lotus seeds and *shatavari*.

HOW TO PREPARE AND USE HERBS ACCORDING TO AYURVEDA

Ayurveda contains many different methods and forms of herbal preparation. All are designed for different therapeutic effects, or to maintain the potencies of herbs in different manners.

These include our standard methods of infusions, decoctions, powders, poultices, oils and liniments, but in a greater variety than generally used in western herbalism. They include herbal wines, jellies, resin preparation, pills and tablets. Other special preparations include minerals, metals, ashes, salts, alkalis and sugars. Preparations are accompanied with *mantra, yantras,* rituals, and fire sacrifices. They are also administered according to certain holy days and along with the phases of the moon and the astrological influences of certain constellations. Confronted with this great abundance, we are limited in our book to the main forms and methods.

THE FIVE MAIN METHODS OF HERBAL PREPARATION
(*Pancha kashaya*)

Raw herbs are generally prepared according to five basic methods of extraction: the fresh juice of the plant (*svarasa*); the crushed pulp or paste of the plant (*kalka*); decoction (*kvatha*); hot infusion (*phant*); and cold infusion (*hima*). Juice is the strongest; cold infusion the weakest. The rest fall into a descending order of strength.

Fresh Juice (*Svarasa*)

The fresh juice of an herb is obtained by taking the fresh plant, crushing or pounding it, then straining the liquid through a cloth. A juicer may also be used for this purpose. This method is not used that often because it relies mainly on freshly picked herbs. Easily available herbs—aloe vera, cilantro, garlic, ginger, lemon, lime, onions, parsley—are also used in the above process, but the effects are best for wild or home grown herbs.

For dry herbs, a weaker juice preparation is made by taking the crushed dry herb or powder, adding twice the weight of the herb in water, allowing to set for 24 hours, and then straining the liquid for a juice substitution.

Herbal Paste (*Kalka*)

The paste of an herb is obtained by crushing the fresh plant—but only to the point where it becomes a soft mass. It can be done with dried herbs, with the addition of enough water to create a workable paste.

Such pastes can be made with honey, ghee or oil, usually in double the amount of the herbs. Various raw sugars can also be used in equal amounts to the herbs. Liquid substances work better with dry herbs, dry substances with fresh herbs.

This mode of preparation is often used externally for plasters and poultices to promote the healing of wounds and sores. (Please see section on Herbs for External Usage.) It may also be used as a basis for infusions and decoctions, an herbal paste being prepared first and then cooked. All herbs can be used in this manner.

Decoction (*Kvatha*)

Herbs are usually administered in the form of a decoction or a hot infusion. The difference is that a decoction involves boiling the herbs over a low flame, while a hot infusion involves cooking them below the boiling point, or steeping them, bringing them to a boil and then removing them from the heat.

The general rule for decoctions: one part dry herbs to sixteen parts water; about half an ounce of herbs per cup or 8 ounces of water. The herbs are then boiled over a low flame until the water is reduced to one quarter of its original amount (for example, four cups would be boiled down to one); the herbs are then strained and the liquid is used as a prepared decoction. This process takes several hours or more and produces a stronger decoction than that usually used in western herbalism.

A moderate decoction, requiring less time, can be made by boiling the herbs until half the water is left. A weak decoction takes even less time to prepare since three-quarters of the water is left. The lesser strength of these preparations can be balanced by taking or giving larger dosages.

The resultant strong tea is then administered usually with other vehicles like honey or hot water (see section on *anupanas* and section on dosages).

In Ayurveda the herbs are only boiled once and then discarded. Some herbalists of other traditions boil them two or three times. This is possible, particularly when the first decoction is of weak or moderate strength.

The decoction method is most suitable for roots, stems, bark and fruit—as harder portions of the plant require longer cooking to release their essence.

Hot Infusion (*Phant*)

For infusions the ratio of herbs to water is one to eight. For example, one ounce herbs per eight ounce cup of water. In the hot infusion, the herbs are added to boiling water and allowed to set for a period of up to twelve hours. This again is longer than the required time used in western herbalism. Usually thirty minutes of steeping is the minimum required for an infusion. The herbs are then strained and the liquid used.

Infusion is better for more delicate plant parts; leaves and flowers, or more herbaceous (non-woody) plants. It is also better for aromatic herbs, like most spices, because boiling destroys and dissipates the aromatic oil.

However, many of these herbs can be cooked below the boiling point over a low flame for a long period of time. This may be necessary in formulas that combine root herbs with flowers or leaves; otherwise the more delicate herbs can be added at a later stage of the decoction.

Cold Infusion (*Hima*)

Cold infusion requires letting the herbs stand in cold water. Usually more time is required for this than for a hot infusion—at least an hour. It is also best to let the herbs stand overnight. This method is necessary for delicate and aromatic herbs, particularly those with cooling energy or refrigerant properties. Cold infusion is best for cooling therapy and reducing high *Pitta* conditions. Such herbs as hibiscus, jasmine, mint and sandalwood are prepared in this manner.

The infusion method is usually best for powders, as they release their properties more quickly than raw herbs. Cold infusion is better for anti-*Pitta* action; otherwise hot infusion is usually best.

ADDITIONAL METHODS OF HERBAL PREPARATION

Milk Decoctions

Decoctions can be done with milk as well as water. The classical method was to take one part herbs, eight parts of milk and thirty-two parts water. The mixture was boiled over a low flame until all the water evaporated. For example, one ounce of herbs was used with one cup of milk and four cups of water.

However, it is also true that smaller amounts of water can be used with certain herbs cooked directly in the milk. This simpler, direct milk decoction can be done with powders. Milk augments the tonic and nutritive effects of herbs, like *ashwagandha* or *shatavari*. It also possesses demulcent properties and combines well with herbs (e.g. comfrey root or slippery elm), for soothing the mucous membranes. It is cooling, helps stop bleeding and reduces inflammation. It can also help to harmonize or work as an antidote in the presence of hot, pungent herbs. Milk may be used as a sedative and it can be combined with certain herbs like gotu kola or nutmeg to promote sleep.

Vessels to Use

According to Ayurveda, the best kind of vessel or pot to use for herbal preparations is an earthen pot. Earthenware combines naturally with herbs the same way plants are intrinsically a part of the soil.

Ayurveda is not, however, opposed to the use of certain metallic vessels, if their properties are understood. For reducing *Kapha*, herbs can be prepared in a copper pot because copper has a scraping and reducing action. For *Pitta* conditions, a pot of brass or silver may be used; these metals are cooling. For *Vata*, iron may be used as it is heavy and grounding. Aluminum should never be used because it will be absorbed in the body as a poison.

Preparing the herbs over a flame, rather than electrical heat, also helps increase their potency and renders them more assimilable to our *Agni*; wood heat is best.

Powders (*Churna*)

Powders are commonly used in Ayurveda. They were tradionally pre-pared with a mortar and pestle and filtered through linen, but they can also be ground mechanically with an herb grinder.

Powders are often easier to make for compounds that consist of many ingredients (Ayurvedic compounds may have twenty or more herbs). Many traditional compounds can be acquired or prepared in the form of powders. They are a simpler mode of preparation than pills or tablets, and can easily be done by herbal practitioners.

Another major advantage of powders is that they require a lower dos-age than raw herbs (one-quarter to one-half), because they allow more of the herb to be ingested directly. Their disadvantage is that their strength diminishes more rapidly, losing potency in six months to one year. How-ever, Ayurvedic powders are prepared by special methods that allow them to last for years.

Powders are not taken by themselves, but with a medium (see *anupanas*). When *ghee*, oil, honey or raw sugar are used, they should be twice the amount of the powder. When milk or water is the vehicle, it should be four times the amount of powder. Bitter powders are usually taken in capsules or with honey.

Powders usually have quick but short term action. They work mainly on the gastrointestinal tract and *rasa dhatu* or plasma. Some rejuvenative herbs, like *ashwagandha, pippali* and *triphala*, which work on all *dhatus*, can be taken as powders.

Pills and Tablets (*Guti* and *Vati*)

Ayurvedic pharmacies offer a wide variety of pills and tablets, often prepared from decoctions.

Gugguls

Guggul (see the herb) is a tree resin very similar to myrrh. Special Ayurvedic pills are made with *guggul*. These are used largely for nervous disorders, for arthritic condition and for weight reduction.

Medicated Wines (*Asavas and Arishtas*)

Ayurveda uses a variety of herbal wines. A yeast culture is added to herbs—either their fresh juice (*arishta*) or their decoction (*asava*) and allowed to ferment for a period of days or months. Often spices are included in this mixture. The resultant herbal wines are easier to assimilate and promote *Agni*. Their properties increase, rather than decrease with aging.

Medicated Jellies (*Avalehas*)

Also used are various herbal jellies or confections. Many tonics and rejuvenatives can be prepared with raw sugar or honey. *Chyavan prash*, a good general tonic (see *amalaki*), is prepared in this way.

Rasa Preparations

There are special Ayurvedic alchemical preparations using humanized forms of mercury, sulphur and other metals. Called *rasa* preparations, they are important in *Rasayan* or rejuvenation therapy and have a powerful action on the nervous system. Other special mineral and metal preparations are used (often in the form of specially incinerated ashes or *bhasma*, which renders them non-toxic to the body.) They are combined with herbs according to the same science of energetics.

All these are more specialized pharmaceutical medicines that are only to be used with the right knowledge. Hopefully, they will become available for Ayurvedic practitioners in this country.

MEDICATED OILS (*Siddha Taila*)

Medicated oils are made by preparing herbs in various oils. Generally, sesame oil is used unless otherwise specified. Other oil-bearing seeds, like coconut, sunflower or castor beans may sometimes be used. Medicated oils are mainly for external use, as in massage, but occasionally they may be taken internally as well.

Medicated oils work on the *dhatus* of *rasa*, *rakta* and *mamsa*, thus increasing the plasma, blood and muscle tissues of the body. They increase the *agnis*, the digestive capacities, of these different tissues. They are too heavy for the liver to digest, and so cannot reach the deeper tissues through it. They work primarily on the skin, blood, lungs and colon. However, through the colon they can have some effect on nerve tissue (*majja dhatu*).

PREPARATION: The main mode of preparation for medicated oils is similar to decoctions. One part of herbs is cooked along with four parts of oil and sixteen parts of water, over a low flame for a period of four to eight hours, until all the water evaporates (when a drop of water placed in the oil makes a crackling sound). For example, two ounces of herbs may be used along with one cup of oil and four cups of water, to make one cup of medicated oil.

Alternately, one can first make the decoction of herbs by itself. Then equal parts of the decoction and the oil are used, and the mixture is similarly cooked until all the decoction evaporates. This method is helpful where one wishes to not include the herbs in the oil—in which case the decoction is strained before being added to the oil.

Some herbs can be added directly to the oil and prepared without water. Aromatic herbs sensitive to heat, like mint, jasmine or camphor, can be added as a powder directly to the oil, one part herbs to four parts oil. The mixture is allowed to stand for 24 to 48 hours, after which it may be strained and is then ready for use.

Other not-quite-as-sensitive aromatic herbs, like cayenne, cloves or mustard, can be added directly to the oil, but they should be cooked over a low flame for several hours, then they may be strained and used.

Fresh juice of herbs, like garlic or ginger juice, may be added in equal amounts to the oil (as in decoctions), and similarly be cooked until all water evaporates. Special care must be taken not to overboil them.

USAGE: Oils may be applied for massage, as ointments for eyes or ears, as dressing for wounds or ulcers, in oil enemas (*basti*), vaginal douches, nasally (*nasya*), and some may be taken orally.

Externally, medicated oils may be good for any of the three *doshas*. Anti-*Pitta* herbs are good in oils for inflammatory conditions of the skin and blood. They are useful in hair loss, premature greying, etc., and may be prepared with coconut oil (which is cooling, while sesame oil is heating).

Anti-*Vata* herbs are good in oils for enemas. Bathing the head in oils (*siro-basti, siro-dhara*) is good for many problems of the brain and nervous system, as well as for diabetes. Oils as *nasya* have a similar usage. Internally, they work mainly on *Vata* and may aggravate *Pitta* and *Kapha*.

Typical herbs used Ayurvedically in medicated oils: *amalaki*, asafoetida, *bala, bhringaraj*, calamus, camphor, garlic, ginger, gotu kola, haritaki, jasmine, mint, *pippali*, saffron, sandalwood, *shatavari*, turmeric, wild indigo.

MEDICATED Ghee (*Siddha Ghrita*)

Medicated ghee is similar to medicated oil. To prepare the ghee itself, heat one pound of raw, unsalted butter on a medium fire for approximately 15 minutes. The butter will melt and start to boil. As it boils, broth will rise to the surface. Do not remove this foam for it contains medicinal properties. Turn the fire to low. The butter will then turn a golden yellow color and will smell rather like popcorn. When a drop or two of water placed in the ghee produces a crackling sound, the ghee is ready. Let it cool slightly and then pour it through a strainer into a container. Ghee may be stored without refrigeration.

The properties and usages of ghee are different than those of medicated oils. Ghee enhances *Ojas*, the subtle essence of all tissues. It increases *Agni* (and all the *agnis*), and all digestive energies and enzymes of the body. It promotes *jatharagni*, the digestive fire dwelling in the small intestine, increasing its capacity without aggravating *Pitta*. It promotes the *bhutagnis*, the elemental fires which dwell in the liver and govern the transformation of food in the body. It does not clog the liver, as do other oils and fats, but strengthens it.

It is food for *majja-dhatu*, bone marrow and nerve tissue, and feeds the brain. Promoting *Ojas*, ghee promotes all the subtle tissues of the body, including *shukra-dhatu*, the reproductive tissues. Through *Ojas* it gives sustenance to *Tejas*, the fire of the mind, and thus promotes *medhagni*, the flame of intelligence and perception. As such, it is an important rejuvenative tonic or *rasayana* for the mind, the brain and the nervous system. It is good for *Vata* and *Pitta doshas*.

For *Pitta* disorders ghee is prepared with bitter herbs. It is similarly prepared for fever, for which ghee is said to be the best medicine.

Ghee is excellent for diseases of the subtle tissues, nerves and mind, including many *Vata* problems.

It is usually taken internally and is often used as *nasya*.

Typical herbs prepared in ghee: bitter herbs generally, *amalaki, ashwagandha, bhringaraj,* calamus, garlic, *gokshura,* gotu kola, jasmine, licorice, *manjishta,* pomegranate, *shatavari, triphala.*

MEDIA OF INTAKE (*Anupana*)

In Ayurveda, herbal medicines are prescribed to be taken with various mediums of intake, as hot water or milk. Such vehicles for taking herbs are called *anupanas.*

Anupanas may enhance the therapeutic effects of herbs. For instance, dry ginger given with honey increases its power of expectoration. Anupanas may relieve the side-effects of herbs, as when hot spices are given with milk to lessen the aggravation of *Pitta.* They may serve as flavoring agents to make medicines palatable. They are used much like supplementary herbs in the formulas themselves.

They can also serve as catalytic agents, or *yogavahis,* to help direct the effects of the herbs to the deeper and subtler tissues of the body. This is the case when ghee is used as an *anupana.*

Anupanas may change the dosha the herbs work on. Ghee is the strongest substance in helping herbs reduce *Pitta* and fever; sesame oil for the reduction of *Vata;* and honey for the reduction of *Kapha.* The same medicine taken with ghee may reduce *Pitta,* but with honey may target *Kapha.*

The simplest way to use *anupanas* is with hot and cold water. Hot water is best for herbs to reduce *Vata* and *Kapha.* Cold water is best to reduce *Pitta.*

However, fever-reducing herbs should always be taken with hot water. Cold water and cold food are contraindicated during fever. It is the suppression of the central digestive fire that causes fever by spreading its heat to the surface of the body. Intake of cold substances supresses it further. Thirst and desire for cold drinks during fever should be relieved by cold sponge baths and warm teas.

Water conveys the effects of herbs to *rasa,* the plasma. Honey brings them to the blood and the muscles. Milk brings them to the plasma and blood. Alcohol brings them to the subtle tissue, to the nerves.

Raw sugar can be used as an *anupana* also. It increases the tonic effect of herbs, much like milk does. It tonifies plasma and blood, relieves heat and protects the tissues, aiding in metabolism.

Typical *anupanas* include: cold water, hot water, honey, *ghee*, butter, raw sugar, herbal decoctions or infusions (like ginger or mint tea), fruit juices, meat soup.

HERBS FOR EXTERNAL USAGE

Many herbs have value in external usage—in washes, pastes, poultices and oils. These herbs can be spoken of as vulneraries, for promoting healing of sores or wounds. It is important that we differentiate their functions and their appropriate times of usage.

Many astringents are famous as vulneraries (see astringent herbs). This is because they promote the knitting of tissues by drying and contracting action. They also have anti-inflammatory properties because of their cooling energy. Many sweet herbs have vulnerary usage (see expectorant and demulcent herbs). This is largely because they have a soothing and softening effect upon the skin and provide nourishment to damaged tissues. Again, they have some anti-inflammatory effects by their cooling energy.

Many bitter herbs are used externally. This is because of their strong anti-inflammatory action, their very cold nature, their refrigerant action on burns, their antiseptic or antibacterial action, and their power to reduce fever. A lot of pungent herbs are used externally because they promote local circulation, ripen boils and promote suppuration. They also provide a counter-irritant action that may be analgesic.

In the initial, acute and often febrile phase of a sore or wound, bitter herbs are most appropriate. When the fever is down and pus formation has begun, pungent herbs are more appropriate. When healing has begun and most pus has been dispelled, astringent (and later sweet) herbs can be used to finalize the healing process. Chronic sores that do not heal may first require the application of pungent herbs to increase local circulation.

Herbs for internal usage in these conditions will be largely the same as those for external usage.

Pungent herbs may be irritating to open sores and to mucous membranes. They are often effective as pastes for relieving pain and headaches.

Herbs for external usage: chickweed, comfrey, flaxseed, Irish moss, licorice, marshmallow, plantain, self-heal, slippery elm, yarrow (all mainly sweet or astringent), asafoetida, barberry, burdock, calamus, ginger, gotu kola, juniper berries, myrrh, sandalwood, sarsaparilla, turmeric, yellow dock.

ROUTES OF ADMINISTRATION

The main route of administration for herbal medicines is through the mouth. Yet other places have their special value.

ENEMA TREATMENT: When the *dosha*, particularly *Vata*, is accumulated in the colon, rectal administration is the preferred route, with medicated enemas (*basti*).

Pungent herbs can be taken this way to clear congestion, mucus and *ama* from the colon. Oils and sweet, moistening herbs can be taken for their lubricating action or for their nutritive effects. Sweet, astringent and bitter herbs can be taken this way for inflammation or ulcerative conditions of the colon. Diuretic herbs can be taken this way. Because of their proximity to the kidneys in enema usage, diuretic herbs can have a very direct effect.

Nasal Administration/Smoking of Herbs

Problems relating to *Prana*, to the nervous and respiratory systems, are often best treated through nasal administration (*nasya*), which includes application of oil to the ears. Snuffing of powders, application of oil to nasal membranes, inhalation of vapors/incense, and taking liquid preparations through the nose to clear the sinuses, are all ways of nasal application.

Pungent herbs, like bayberry or ginger, can be taken this way for their clearing and decongestant action. Nervines (like gotu kola) may be taken this way, particularly as a medicated *ghee*, (taken in 5 drops in each nostril, lying down), for direct action on the brain.

Also included in nasal administration is the smoking of herbs. Herbs are often smoked as part of detoxification therapy (after *pancha karma*) to burn residual toxins from the system. Herbs may also be used in the place of tobacco to help stop smoking.

Smoking of herbs helps enhance their decongestant and anti-cough action and is good for colds and sore throats. It gives them immediate action on the nerves and may help clear the mind for yoga and meditation.

Herbs for smoking: *ajwan*, bayberry, black pepper, cardamom, cinnamon, cloves, cubebs, ginger (mainly hot, pungent, expectorants) and such special rejuvenatives for the mind as calamus and gotu kola.

Eye Administration

Problems relating to *vyana*, the *vata* that governs muscular movement and the circulatory system, may be treated through herbal medicines applied to the eyes (*anjana*). Herbs to restore a patient to consciousness can be given this way, as well as herbs for local eye problems. Under this are also included eye drops, oils for the eyes, and ointments applied in and around the eyes.

Skin Administration

Application of herbs and oils to the skin is another major route. This is helpful not only for local skin problems, but can help in many other conditions, including different *Vata* disorders, weakness of the lungs and the nervous system. Massage with herbal oils is one of the best means of reducing high *Vata*.

Special oil administration may involve the use of *ghee* or sesame oil on the sites of the seven *chakras*, either on the back or the front of the body. For example, high *Pitta* can often be reduced by the application of sandalwood oil at the site of the third eye.

Like Chinese medicine, Ayurveda recognizes the value of heating special meridian points on the body. Called moxibustion in the Chinese system, it is called *Agni karma*, fire-treatment, in Ayurveda.

Ayurveda uses turmeric, calamus, or metallic rods, usually copper or silver, heated and superficially applied to vital points or *chakras*. This helps burn toxins and stimulate organ function. The herbs may be made into a cigarette and burned about half an inch above the points to be treated, until they become hot.

TIMES OF ADMINISTRATION

Ayurveda recognizes that the times of taking herbs are important in strengthening their effects.

A good simple general rule to follow is that herbs taken before meals, a half-hour to an hour, tend to work on the colon and the lower part of the body, on *apana vayu*, the air or *Vata* governing eliminatory functions.

Herbs taken with the meal tend to work on the stomach and small intestine, on the middle part of the body and *samana vayu*, the air governing digestive functions. And herbs taken after meals tend to work on the lungs, on the upper part of the body and on *prana vayu*, the air governing respiratory functions.

Herbs that tend to work on the lower part of the body, such as purgatives, diuretics and emmenagogues, and herbs targeting the colon, the kidneys or the reproductive organs, should be taken before meals. Herbs working on digestive functions (stimulants and carminatives, bitter tonics, or nutritive tonics, which are taken like food), and herbs that target the stomach, spleen, liver or small intestine, should be taken with meals. Herbs that tend to work on the upper part of the body—diaphoretics, expectorants, nervines—and herbs that target the lungs, heart or brain, should be taken after meals.

Other times of administration are discriminated

Rejuvenatives are often taken first thing in the morning, as are herbs that reduce *Kapha* and mucus.

Strong purgatives may be taken first thing in the morning for those who rise early, or just before sleep for those who have to be at work early in the morning.

Some herbs are taken before bed, an hour before sleep; this is particularly true of herbs for insomnia or other sleep disorders.

At meals, a little of an herb may be taken with every morsel of food. This works with strong medications, for those who have difficulty getting herbs down, and when using herbs (hot spices) that increase *Agni*.

Herbs may be taken between meals to help in the increase of metabolism.

Herbs can also be taken moment by moment, for acute conditions like *Prana* disturbances of asthma, vomiting and hiccough.

Generally speaking, strong medicines are given during acute attacks and weaker medication between attacks, and for chronic conditions.

COMPOUNDS

In Ayurveda, herbs are generally not used alone but in compounds. Ayurveda holds that the right combination of herbs greatly increases their healing powers, helps expand the field of their activity and compensates for their side effects. To the understanding of the qualities of individual herbs should be added the art of combining them, the Ayurvedic yoga of their usage. There are laws and principles in constructing compounds through which they can be formulated and understood.

In combining herbs, first of all it is necessary to select an individual herb that best represents the healing actions most appropriate for the individual person and his or her condition, as with a prime diaphoretic like bayberry to treat the common cold.

To this should be added herbs of similar properties. The main principle behind all compounds is that herbs of similar properties enhance each other. An equal amount of a combination of similar herbs has a stronger therapeutic effect than the same amount of any one herb by itself. For example, in the compound *trikatu*, consisting of dry ginger, black pepper and *pippali* (Indian long pepper), in which all three herbs promote digestion and assimilation, 500 mg. of this compound has a much stronger effect than 500 mg. of any single one of these herbs.

Herbs often have more than one action. Which will be their main action will depend upon the herbs with which they are combined. For example, combined with diaphoretic herbs like bayberry or ephedra, the diaphoretic action of cinnamon is activated and enhanced. Combined with digestive agents like cardamom or bay leaves, it will have an action more on that level.

Apart from a few herbs that share the main action of the primary herb in a formula, a few herbs which share related actions may be added as assistants. In a diaphoretic or sweating formula to relieve a cold or flu, some other herbs may be added for such related problems as cough or to dispel mucus.

Besides this synergistic action of similar herbs there is the antidotal action of contrary herbs. Often a formula may contain an herb or two whose action is opposite that of the majority of herbs contained in it. Such antidotal herbs serve to balance out the formula and prevent it from having too excessive or one-sided an action. They alleviate potential side-effects and may have a protective action on the tissues.

Formulas that contain very hot herbs like cloves or *pippali,* according to this principle, may also contain some raw sugar or rock candy. This has an opposite cooling property, which makes them easier to take.

In formulas that aim at purification some tonic herbs may be included for their protective action. In formulas that aim at tonification, some light digestive herbs may be included to counter their tendency, by their heaviness, to weaken digestion.

In addition to these major herbs in a formula, some other herbs may be added in small dosages to facilitate their usage by the body. Compounds may contain some stimulant herbs to aid in the absorption and assimilation of the other herbs in the formulas. In western herbalism, cayenne pepper is generally used in this capacity, or sometimes dry ginger. In Ayurveda, the compound *trikatu* is usually used. Such substances are called *prakshepa dravyas,* or means of energization. More developed formulas may contain five or more of these substances, but their dosage is small enough so that they insure the main herbs are properly digested without changing their action.

An herb or two may further be added as eliminators, so that there is not a build-up of toxins or waste-materials. Even tonic formulas may have such herbs, which are largely diuretics or laxatives. This is why many Ayurvedic formulas contain the compound *triphala,* a laxative, in small dosages.

Finally formulas may include or be taken with substances to serve as mediums for directing their effects to the deeper tissues (like honey, see *anupanas*).

In this way, with our main herb and its strengtheners as the major ingredients, various assistant and counter-assistant herbs are added as secondary agents. Then certain stimulants and eliminators are added for additional enhancement and the whole formula is taken with certain carrier substances to give it maximum effect. Making compounds is an art that requires practice. One should start off simply.

DOSAGES
Traditional Dosages for Medical Usage

Decoction

1. Strong: Take 4 ounces of herbs in 1/2 gallon of water. Boil over a low flame until the liquid is reduced to 1 pint (16 fluid ounces). Dosage is 1/4 cup (2 fluid ounces), 3 times a day.

2. Moderate: take 4 ounces of herbs in 1 quart of water. Boil over a low flame until liquid is reduced to 1 pint. Same dosage.

Infusion

1. Strong: Add 4 ounces of herbs to 1 pint of boiling water. Allow to set for at least 3 hours. Dosage 1/4 cup 3 times a day.

2. Moderate: Add 2 ounces of herbs to 1 pint boiling water. Allow to set for at least 3 hours. Same dosage.

For cold infusion follow the same procedure, but add herbs to cold water.

Powder

1. High dosage, 3 to 6 grams 3 times a day.

2. Low dosage: 1/2 to 3 grams.

Anupana

Medical dosages should be given with suitable *anupana* (see *anupanas.*) The simplest way is equal amounts of hot water to each herbal preparation.

Temperature

Infusions and decoctions should be taken hot; powders should be taken along with a warm *anupana*, except in *Pitta* conditions where there is no fever. In feverish conditions, herbs should also be taken hot.

Caution

Ayurveda has no standard dosage of medicines. Its dosages depend upon the age of the person, body weight, strength of digestion, constitution, as well as strength and duration of the disease. To give standard dosages is a simplification that may be misleading. When in doubt, use lower dosages, increasing until the proper effect is realized.

These strong dosages of herbs are usually given in compounds, and balanced to relieve possible side-effects of the herbs, to ensure their proper assimilation. These compounds consist of from three to fifty herbs. If a single herb is being prepared in these dosages, it is best to follow moderate or low dosage.

Dosage for Common Usage

Large dosages should only be used when the right knowledge and expertise are present, preferably when prescribed by a qualified practitioner.

For common usage these lower dosages and weaker preparations should be used, as follows:

1. Infusion: 1 teaspoon (3 grams) per cup. Let steep for 30 minutes.

2. Decoction: 2 teaspoons (6 grams) per cup. Let boil over a low flame for 30 minutes. The same for milk decoctions.

3. Powder: 2 "00" capsules or about 1 gram.

Most dosages will be taken three times a day. As herb weights vary considerably, please use a scale when possible.

Note

Herbs that are very hot and pungent, like cayenne, or very cold and bitter, like golden seal, should always be used in low dosages, while those that are sweet or heavy, like comfrey root, should generally be used in high dosages. A good general rule is to use light, strong tasting herbs in less than one-half the normal dosage; heavy, bland tasting herbs should be used in double the standard dosage.

DIAGRAM 6   *Shri Yantra*

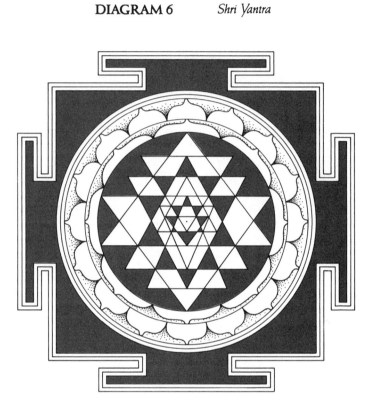

MANTRA, YANTRA AND MEDITATION

There are two levels of healing in Ayurveda: the physical and the mental. The basic means of healing on the physical level is through herbs. The basic means of healing on the mental or psychological level is through *mantras*. *Mantras* are special seed syllables like *Om* which reflect the cosmic creative vibration. The plant transmits the seed-energy of nature into the body; the *mantra* transmits the seed-energy of the spirit into the mind.

These two levels of healing are always related. Plants have their effects upon the mind, and *mantras* change our physiology. Both work on the *Prana* or life-force—one from without, the other from within. The human being, as mentioned earlier, is the essence of plants. The essence of the human being is speech, the essence of which is the *mantra*. In harmony with the plant as the word of nature is the *mantra*, the word of the spirit. Between these stands the human being.

The mind is refined through plants. In the *mantra* it is perfected. Hence, the right use of herbs and a vegetarian diet serve as catalysts for the *mantric* development of consciousness. This is the beauty of Ayurveda — that it is not limited to the "normal" idea of physical health, but shows us how to incorporate healing into the practice of yoga and the liberation of the spirit. In doing this, the *mantra* becomes the means of directing the healing energy of plants into the mind. It gives herbs a power of psychological healing and spiritual integration. It brings the universal intelligence of nature into harmony with the individual.

All plants and all healing processes have certain *mantric* affinities. All plants, all life is a manifestation of the *mantra*, which is the structuring power of the cosmic mind. Through the *mantra* all things are empowered.

Without the use of *mantra*, which means the right energization of the mind, any healing process remains outward and superficial. With the right use of the *mantra*, which means the giving of right attention, the healing process becomes a conscious act, and thereby a means of healing consciousness.

Mantra is not merely a matter of mechanically repeating various powerful sounds. *Mantra* also implies meditation. Meditation (*dhyana*), means receptivity, passive awareness, in which there is the unity of the seer and the seen. It means understanding, the attitude of openness in which there is space for the inner truth to manifest itself. This inner truth that comes from all things in meditation is itself the *mantra*. The true power of *mantra* appears in meditation. The right use of *mantra* implies establishing the healing space of meditation.

Plants meditate. The earth meditates. The sun vibrates the great *mantra Om* as it moves in the sky. All of nature is the creative meditation of the cosmic spirit. The basic silence and peace of nature is meditation.

It is much too complicated here to discuss specific *mantras*, which relate to specific therapies, but there is one great *mantra* through which all herbal preparations can be energized. It is the great *mantra* of the Goddess.

The Goddess (*Devi*) is the *Shakti*, the divine energy working in nature, through which all healing, integration and evolution proceed. She, the Divine Mother, prepares the right food and medicine for all life forms. It is only through her that our food and medicine has nourishing and healing power. Therefore, giving power to her in the *mantra* energizes all things accordingly.

This *mantra* is *OM AIM HRIM KLIM CHAMUNDAYAI VICCHE* (pronounced *om aim hreem kling chamoondayee vichay*). It is the *mantra* to the Goddess *Chamunda*, who integrates within herself the three great Goddesses of *Saraswati*, *Durga* and *Kali*, along with their three elements of air, fire and water (*Vata*, *Pitta* and *Kapha*), and their three centers of the head, the navel, and the base of the spine.

Doing this *mantra* 108 times while preparing herbal medicines, or upon taking them, will give them a greatly increased potency. Originally, Ayurvedic medicines were prepared with a *mantra*. Just as food should be prepared with love to be really nourishing, so herbs should be prepared with a *mantra*. It is not what we prepare, but how we prepare it. All healing practices should flow from the love and the awareness of a *mantra*.

Along with *mantra* comes *yantra*. *Mantra* is the seed-syllable of the cosmic creative vibration; *yantra* is the pattern it creates, its energy field. *Mantra* is the name of the deity; *yantra* is the subtle form. *Yantras* are mystic diagrams, geometrical designs that manifest cosmic law (which, in more complicated designs, become mandalas).

Yantras are drawn on silk, on the bark of certain trees, on copper and on gold (copper is usually best for most purposes). Ayurvedic medicines are often prepared with *yantras* or in the presence of a *yantra*. *Yantras*, which are largely composed of triangular or pyramid shapes, serve to draw in the cosmic life force and establish a space for healing to occur. With the *mantra* they purify the astral aura and cleanse the psychic environment, which is always impure or stagnant in the case of disease.

Yantras can also be used to purify food or water, to potentize (increase the power and depth of penetration) medicines, as well as to purify the treatment room. They can be placed on certain parts of the body, like the *chakras*, to release blockages. In this regard they can be used in conjunction with crystals and gem-stones.

We have illustrated the *Shri Yantra*, which is the king of the *yantras*, the great *yantra* of the goddess that represents and contains within itself the entire universe. This *yantra* goes with the *mantra* to the goddess and can be used generally for all forms of healing and preparation of herbs.

HERBS FOR AYURVEDIC USAGE

The first section of our herb list consists of typical western herbs and their Ayurvedic usage. Emphasis has been on herbs used both in India as well as the west, and so a number of common spices have been selected. The attempt has been to include a variety of herbs in different categories. Owing to the limitation of space, other valuable herbs could not be so explicated. These are given, with their more basic indication, in the appendix.

The first name of the herb is its English or most commonly known name. Second is the Latin name and plant family. Third is the Sanskrit (S) name and fourth is the Chinese (C) name, when available.

Energetics are taste (*rasa*), energy (*virya*), and post-digestive effect (*vipaka*). V is *Vata*, P is *Pitta*, K is *Kapha*; + or − are increases or decreases. VPK = is balancing to all three *doshas*. *Ama* is toxins.

Tissues are the Ayurvedic *dhatus*; systems relate to the Ayurvedic *srotas*.

The second section consists of some major oriental herbs. It includes important Indian herbs not commonly known here yet (a few are available through Indian markets). It also includes some Chinese herbs, like ginseng, that are becoming popular here and may be used like Ayurvedic tonics, particularly when the latter are not available. Some of the herbs in this section are used both in Indian and Chinese medicine. Emphasis has been on tonic and rejuvenative herbs, for which there are not always substitutes in available western herbs. Many other important Indian herbs exist. Only a few major ones have been given by way of example.

Tastes, when multiple, and actions, are usually in descending order of strength.

Dosage and preparation of herbs will generally be according to our section on dosage. The more specific dosages given for individual herbs will be based on common usage.

Powders of all herbs can be prepared as infusions. (Decoctions are for harder and heavier raw herbs, like most roots.)

Indications of conditions treated by the herbs are suggestive rather than exhaustive. Precautions are not necessarily contraindications. The same disease condition may occur in different forms and so require different treatment and have different contraindications.

Ayurvedic treatment is to cleanse the body of *Ama*, balance the constitution and promote rejuvenation. It does not treat diseases as specific entities but as by-products of aggravated *doshas*.

A. COMMONLY AVAILABLE HERBS

ALFALFA   *Medicago sativa; Leguminosae*

Part Used: herb
Energetics: astringent, sweet/cooling/pungent
      PK– V+
Tissues: plasma, blood
Systems: circulatory, urinary
Actions: alterative, diuretic, antipyretic, hemostatic
Indications: ulcers, edema, arthritis, vitamin or mineral deficiency
Precautions: high *Vata*
Preparation: infusion, powder (250 mg to 1 g)

ALFALFA is a natural mineral and vitamin supplement. It contains organic minerals like calcium, magnesium, phosphorus and potassium, and almost all known vitamins. It is also very high in chlorophyll. As such, it combines well with other natural supplements like dandelion, horsetail, nettles and parsley.

However, it is not entirely tonic or nutritive in the Ayurvedic sense, for by itself it does not really provide substance for building tissue. Its action is cleansing and detoxifying. It has a drying effect that may aggravate *Vata*, increasing emaciation. For such individuals, it is best taken occasionally or as balanced out by more nutritive tonics.

It is a mild blood purifier and a good general beverage for *Pitta* (and also, to a lesser degree, *Kapha*) constitutions.

ALOE   *Aloe spp.; Liliaceae*

(S) *Kumari*, a young girl or virgin; aloe is so called because it imparts the energy of youth and brings about the renewal of the female nature.

(C) Lu hui

Part Used: gel (fresh or powdered)
Energetics: bitter, astringent, pungent, sweet/cooling/sweet
        VPK = (gel), powder except in very low dosages will
        aggravate V
Tissues: works on all tissues
Systems: circulatory, digestive, female reproductive, excretory
Actions: alterative, bitter tonic, rejuvenative, emmenagogue, purgative, vulnerary
Indications: fever, constipation, obesity, inflammatory skin conditions, swollen glands, conjunctivitis, bursitis, jaundice, hepatitis, enlarged liver or spleen, herpes, venereal diseases, amenorrhea, dysmenorrhea, menopause, vaginitis, tumors, intestinal worms
Precautions: pregnancy, uterine bleeding
Preparation: fresh gel, powder (100 to 500 mg)

ALOE gel is a wonderful tonic for the liver and spleen, for the blood and the female reproductive system. Aloe regulates sugar and fat metabolism and tonifies all the *agnis*, the digestive enzymes of the body; and at the same time it reduces *Pitta*. It is rejuvenative for *Pitta* and for the uterus. Two teaspoons of it can be taken three times a day, with a pinch of turmeric, as a general tonic. It is more palatable mixed with water or apple juice. Or three ounces of the gel can be taken from a fresh plant along with three ounces of water, three teaspoons of salt, brought to a boil and combined with one ounce of raw sugar and taken in teaspoonful doses. Commercial aloe juices are often diluted and combined with other additives that may give them a different effect.

As a nutritive tonic, aloe can be combined with *shatavari*, as a bitter tonic with gentian, and as an alterative and emmenagogue with *manjishta*. The fresh juice can be applied externally for burns, sores, herpes, etc.

Aloe powder is a powerful laxative that must be used in small
amounts. The powder's taste is nauseating and so it should be taken in
capsules. The powder can also cause severe griping and should be
taken with a carminative herb like turmeric or rose flowers.

DIAGRAM 7   Plant- Aloe

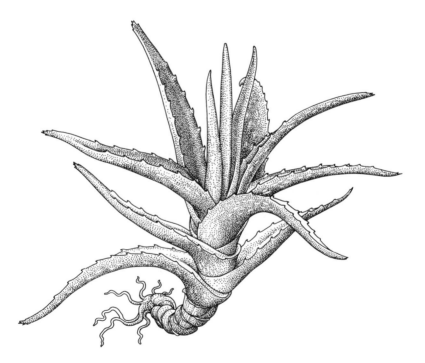

BARBERRY   *Berberis spp.; Berberidaceae*

(S) *Daruharidra,* wood turmeric, owing to its similar properties to turmeric

Part Used: root
Energetics: bitter, astringent/heating/pungent
        PK– V+
Tissues: plasma, blood, fat
Systems: circulatory, digestive
Actions: bitter tonic, alterative, antipyretic, laxative, anthelmintic, bacteriocidal, amoebicidal
Indications: fever (remittent and intermittent), enlargement of liver and spleen, conjunctivitis, acne, boils, chronic dysentery (amoebic, bacillary), jaundice, hepatitis, diabetes
Precautions: high *Vata,* tissue deficiency
Preparation: decoction, powder (250 mg to 1 g), medicated *ghee,* paste

BARBERRY is a bitter herb with a special heating potency (*prabhava*), which is its special property to destroy *Ama* or toxins in the body. Generally speaking, it can be treated like other bitter herbs, with its *Pitta*-reducing and *Vata*-increasing attributes. However, in this respect it is less likely to aggravate *Vata* (particularly when combined with turmeric) than other such herbs.

Barberry is specific for cleansing the liver and regulating its function. For reducing *Ama* or fat in the body, it is combined with turmeric. With twice the amount of turmeric it can be used in diabetes. For controlling *Pitta* it can be used with other bitter tonics like golden seal or *nimb* leaves.

BASIL   *Ocinum spp.; Labiatae*

(S) *Tulsi*

Part Used: herb
Energetics: pungent/heating/pungent
        VK– P+ (in excess)
Tissues: plasma, blood, marrow and nerves, reproductive
Systems: respiratory, nervous, digestive

Properties: diaphoretic, febrifuge, nervine, antispasmodic, antibacterial, antiseptic
Actions: colds, cough, sinus congestion, headaches, arthritis, rheumatism, fevers (generally), abdominal distention
Precautions: high *Pitta*
Preparation: infusion, powder (250 mg to 1 g), juice, medicated *ghee*

Next to the Lotus, BASIL is perhaps the most sacred plant of India. Its quality is pure *Sattva*. Basil opens the heart and mind, bestowing the energy of love and devotion (*bhakti*). Sacred to *Vishnu* and *Krishna*, it strengthens faith, compassion and clarity. *Tulsi* stems are worn as rosaries and promote the energy of attachment. Basil gives the protection of the divine by clearing the aura and strengthening the immune system. It contains natural mercury, which, as the semen of *Shiva*, gives the seed-power of pure awareness.

A plant of basil should be kept in every house for its purifying influence. Basil absorbs positive ions, energizes negative ions, and liberates ozone from the sun's rays.

Basil is an effective diaphoretic and febrifuge in most colds, flus and lung problems. It removes excess *Kapha* from the lungs and nasal passages, increasing *Prana* and promoting sensory acuity. It also removes high *Vata* from the colon, improves absorption and strengthens the nerve tissue, increasing memory. Basil may be taken as a beverage with honey for promoting clarity of mind.

The fresh leaf juice is used externally for fungal infections on the skin.

BAYBERRY   *Myrica spp.; Myricaceae*

(S) *Katphala*

Part Used: bark, fruit
Energetics: pungent, astringent/heating/pungent KV– P+
Tissues: plasma, blood, marrow and nerve
Systems: respiratory, nervous, circulatory, lymphatic
Actions: diaphoretic, expectorant, astringent, emetic, antispasmodic, alterative

Indications: colds, flus, laryngitis, sinus and nasal congestion, sore throat, asthma, bronchitis, adenoids, fever, bleeding gums, chronic sores, epilepsy
Precautions: high *Pitta*, hyperacidity, hypertension
Preparation: decoction, powder (250 mg to 1 g), paste

BAYBERRY is a powerful anti-*Kapha* medicine. It dispels colds, mucus, cleanses the lymphatics and promotes emesis, all of which subdues high *Kapha*. It improves the voice, opens the mind and senses and clears the sinuses. Bayberry is a primary diaphoretic for colds and flus and works well with cinnamon and ginger. As an effective medicine for sore throats, spongy gums, it may be gargled. It can be "snuffed" nasally or smoked to clear the lungs and sinuses. It decongests *Vata* in the head and strengthens *Prana*. Bayberry promotes the healing of mucous membranes and when used as a paste or wash, it is good for old wounds and sores that do not heal.

Bayberry is sacred to *Shiva* and *Shakti*. Bayberry fruit is offered to *Durga*. The dry skin of the fruit is smoked to help calm the mind and open perception. Its quality is *sattvic*. It is one of the best herbs for the initial stage of diseases and mobilizes the defensive energy of the body.

BLACK PEPPER   *Piper nigrum; Piperaceae*

(S) *Marich*, a name for the sun, owing to its containing large amounts of solar energy

(C) Hu jiao

Part Used: fruit
Energetics: pungent/heating/pungent
          KV– P+
Tissues: plasma, blood, fat, marrow and nerve
Systems: digestive, circulatory, respiratory
Actions: stimulant, expectorant, carminative, febrifuge, anthelmintic
Indications: chronic indigestion, toxins in colon, degenerated metabolism, obesity, sinus congestion, fever, intermittent fever, cold extremities

Precautions: inflammatory conditions of the digestive organs, high *Pitta*

Preparation: infusion, powder (100 to 500 mg), milk decoction, medicated *ghee*

BLACK PEPPER is one of the most powerful digestive stimulants. It burns up *Ama* and cleanses the alimentary canal (energizing *Agni* to destroy toxins and digest food). Black pepper can be taken nasally as a medicated *ghee* to relieve sinus congestion, headaches, and even epileptic seizures. It is a good antidote to cold food like cucumbers and for excessive intake of raw food and salads. Used externally, it helps ripen boils and promote suppuration. Prepared in *ghee*, it heals inflamed surfaces, such as in urticaria and erysipelas. With honey, it is a powerful expectorant and mucus-cleanser, drying up secretions. If used excessively, black pepper can act as an irritant as its quality is *rajasic*.

BURDOCK   *Arctium lappa; Compositae*

(C) Niu bang

Part Used: root and seeds
Energetics: bitter, pungent and astringent (root also sweet)/cooling/pungent PK— V+ (in excess)
Tissues: plasma, blood
Systems: respiratory, urinary, circulatory, lymphatic
Actions: alterative, diaphoretic, diuretic, antipyretic
Indications: inflammatory skin conditions, rashes, cold with fever and sore throat, toxins in the blood, lymphatic clogging, nephritis, edema, kidney inflammation, hypertension
Precautions: anemia, chronic chills, high *Vata*
Preparation: infusion (cold or hot), decoction (root), powder (250 mg to 1 g), paste

BURDOCK has a strong action in cleansing the blood and the lymphatics. It clears congestion, reduces swelling and dispels toxins (either from the skin or through diuresis). Burdock seeds have a strong diuretic and detoxifying action and help relieve cough. Burdock root has more nutritive properties and is less likely to increase *Vata*. It can be considered a tonic and rejuvenative for *Pitta* for use on a regular basis. It is good for helping clear high *Pittogenic* emotions like anger, aggression and ambition.

Burdock can be used in most *Ama* conditions, including toxic fever (*Ama jvara*) and arthritis (*Ama Vata*). Burdock root works well with yellow dock. Burdock seeds can be used with coriander seeds. As a tonic for *Pitta*, burdock root can be combined with *bhringaraj*, in proportions of 2 to 1, respectively.

CALAMUS ROOT (Sweet Flag)   *Acorus calamus; Araceae*

(S) *Vacha*, which means literally "speaking", the power of the word, of intelligence or self-expression that this herb stimulates

(C) Shi chang pu

Part Used: rhizome
Energetics: pungent, bitter, astringent/heating/pungent
          VK– P+
Tissues: plasma, muscle, fat, marrow and nerve, reproductive
Systems: nervous, respiratory, digestive, circulatory, reproductive
Actions: stimulant, rejuvenative, expectorant, decongestant, nervine, antispasmodic, emetic
Indications: colds, cough, asthma, sinus headaches, sinusitis, arthritis, epilepsy, shock, coma, loss of memory, deafness, hysteria, neuralgia
Precautions: bleeding disorders including epistaxis, bleeding hemorrhoids
Preparation: decoction, milk decoction, powder (250 to 500 mg), paste

CALAMUS is currently under F.D.A. restrictions, not recommended for internal usage and held to be toxic. However, it has been used in Ayurveda for many thousands of years, being one of the most reknowned herbs of the ancient *Vedic* seers. It is a rejuvenative for the brain and the nervous system, which it purifies and revitalizes. As such it is also a rejuvenative for *Vata*, and secondarily for *Kapha*. It clears the subtle channels of toxins and obstructions. It promotes cerebral circulation, increases sensitivity, sharpens memory and enhances awareness. It is *sattvic* and one of the best herbs for the mind, along

DIAGRAM 8 Calamus

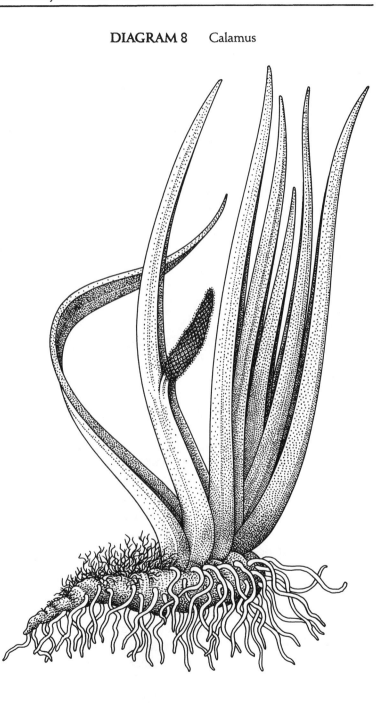

with *brahmi* (gotu kola) for which purposes it can be combined. It also helps transmute sexual energy and feeds *kundalini*.

It can be applied externally as a paste on the forehead for headaches or on painful arthritic joints. It is perhaps the best herb for nasal administration, for nasal congestion and nasal polyps, and it directly revitalizes *Prana*. In large doses it is an emetic. To counter its emetic properties for general usage, it can be taken with equal amounts of fresh ginger, 2 grams each per cup of water, with a little honey.

The powder taken nasally, in small doses, is also a simple and effective restorative to those in shock or coma.

CAMPHOR   *Cinnamomum camphora; Lauraceae*

(S) *Karpura*

(C) Jand

Part Used: crystallized distilled oil
Energetics: pungent, bitter/heating (slightly)/pungent
            KV– P+ (in excess)
Tissues: plasma, blood, fat, marrow and nerve
Systems: respiratory, nervous
Actions: expectorant, decongestant, stimulant, antispasmodic, broncho-dilator, nervine, analgesic, antiseptic
Indications: bronchitis, asthma, whooping cough, pulmonary congestion, hysteria, epilepsy, delirium, insomnia, dysmenorrhea, gout, rheumatism, nasal congestion, sinus headaches, eye problems, tooth decay
Precautions: in excess, camphor acts as a narcotic poison, aggravating *Pitta* and *Vata*; use only in prescribed low dosages
Preparation: infusion (cold, half-ounce crystals to one gallon of water, dosage 2 ounces), powder (100 to 250 mg), medicated oil

CAMPHOR increases *Prana*, opens up the senses and brings clarity to the mind. While in western herbalism it is used only externally as an oil, in Ayurveda it is also taken internally in small dosages in the form of infused or powdered camphor crystals. It is also applied to the eyes in small amounts; though initially burning, it promotes tears and cools and clears the eyes. A pinch of camphor powder is taken nasally for congestion, headache and to awaken perception. It is burned as an incense externally during *Puja*, devotional worship, to purify the atmosphere (its quality is *sattvic*), and promote meditation.

Camphor is perhaps the main herb used in medicated oils throughout the world. It works well in sesame oil: 1 ounce of powder per pint of oil. As such, it is a good stimulant and counter-irritant for joint and muscle pain. Camphor infusion can also be boiled and its vapor inhaled for respiratory application. Use only the raw camphor for internal usage, not the commonly sold synthetic camphor.

CARDAMOM   *Elettaria cardamomum; Zingiberaceae*

(S) *Ela*

(C) Sha ren

Part Used: seed
Energetics: pungent, sweet/heating/pungent
VK– P+ (in excess)
Tissues: plasma, blood, marrow and nerve
Systems: digestive, respiratory, circulatory, nervous
Actions: stimulant, expectorant, carminative, stomachic, diaphoretic
Indications: colds, cough, bronchitis, asthma, hoarse voice, loss of taste, poor absorption, indigestion
Precautions: ulcers, high *Pitta*
Preparation: infusion (do not boil), powder (100 to 500 mg), milk decoction

CARDAMOM is one of the best and safest digestive stimulants. It awakens the spleen, stimulates *samana vayu*, enkindles *Agni* and removes *Kapha* from the stomach and lungs. It stimulates the mind and heart and gives clarity and joy. Added to milk it neutralizes its mucus forming properties and it detoxifies caffein in coffee. Its quality is *sattvic* and it is particularly good for opening and soothing the flow of the *pranas* in the body.

Cardamom is good for the nervous digestive upset of children or of high *Vata* and in this regard combines well with fennel. It helps stop vomiting, belching, or acid regurgitation.

CAYENNE PEPPER   *Capsicum annuum; Solanaceae*

(S) *Marichi-phalam,* fruit of the sun, like black pepper *(marich),* it contains large amounts of solar energy

Part Used: fruit
Energetics: pungent/heating/pungent
            KV– P+
Tissues: plasma, blood, some action on marrow, nerves and reproductive
Systems: digestive, circulatory, respiratory
Actions: Stimulant, diaphoretic, expectorant, carminative, alterative, hemostatic, anthelmintic
Indications: indigestion, *Ama,* poor absorption, abdominal distention, worms, sinus congestion, chronic chill, poor circulation
Precautions: ulcers, gastritis, enteritis, inflammatory conditions of the g.i. tract generally speaking, irritant to mucous membranes
Preparation: infusion, powder (low dosage, 100 to 500 mg)

According to Ayurveda, CAYENNE is not a panacea, though it is a very valuable medicine. It is a strong stimulant, both circulatory and digestive, and a strong dispeller of internal and external cold. It is food for *Agni.* However, cayenne can aggravate inflammatory conditions in the body. Although it is not to be used indiscriminately, it does enhance the properties of many other herbs.

Cayenne has strong hemostatic action and can be used in acute condition to stop bleeding. However, long term usage of cayenne can promote hemorrhaging by its heating property. It is helpful in cases of heart weakness or heart attack for revival purposes, but it can also aggravate high *Pitta,* which causes some heart attacks.

Cayenne can be used with other herbs wherever stimulant action is required. It is particularly effective in burning toxins from the colon. It has similar properties to black pepper but is stronger in short term usage and weaker in long term effect. Its quality is *rajasic* and so it may increase disturbance in the mind if used too much.

CHAMOMILE

Anthemis nobilis (Roman)
Matricaria chamomilla (German);
Compositae

Part Used: flowers, herb
Energetics: bitter, pungent/cooling/pungent
     KP– V+ (in excess)
Tissues: plasma, blood, muscles, marrow and nerve
Systems: respiratory, digestive, nervous
Actions: diaphoretic, carminative, nervine, antispasmodic, analgesic, emmenagogue, emetic
Indications: headaches, indigestion, digestive and nervous problems of children, colic, eye inflammations, jaundice, dysmenorrhea, amenorrhea
Precautions: large dosages are emetic and may aggravate *Vata*
Preparation: infusion (hot or cold), powder (250 to 1 g), paste

CHAMOMILE is a popular beverage tea with many therapeutic values. In moderate amounts it is good for all constitutions, and it is a particularly good beverage for *Pitta*. It helps relieve bilious, digestive headaches, relieves congestion of the blood and promotes menstruation. It is a *sattvic* herb that is very balancing to the emotions. It sedates nerve pain and strengthens the eyes.

A little fresh ginger prepared with it makes chamomile a completely balanced beverage and counters any emetic effect it might have. Externally, it can be used as an eye wash or as a poultice for nerve pains. For most medical purposes its action is mild and serves as a harmonizing adjunct.

CINNAMON

Cinnamomum zeylanicum; Lauraceae

(S) *Twak*

(C) Gui

Part Used: bark
Energetics: pungent, sweet, astringent/heating/sweet
     VK– P+
Tissues: plasma, blood, muscles, marrow and nerves

Systems: circulatory, digestive, respiratory, urinary
Actions: stimulant, diaphoretic, carminative, alterative, expectorant,
diuretic, analgesic
Indications: colds, sinus congestion, bronchitis, dyspepsia
Precautions: high *Pitta*, bleeding disorders
Preparation: infusion, decoction, powder (500 mg to 1 g)

CINNAMON is an effective herb for strengthening and harmonizing
the flow of circulation (*vyana vayu*). It is a good diaphoretic and expectorant in colds and flus, and is especially good for those of weak constitution. It is a pain reliever for toothache and muscle tension. It
strengthens the heart, warms the kidneys and promotes *Agni*. Like ginger, it is almost a universal medicine, and is less likely to aggravate *Pitta*
than ginger. It is a good general beverage (its quality is *sattvic*) for *Vata*
constitution.

It is the basis for the Three Aromatics, along with cardamom and bay
leaves. These three help promote digestion, strengthen *samana vayu*,
and help in the absorption of medicines. They occur together like
Trikatu (dry ginger, black pepper and *pippali*), in many Ayurvedic
formulas.

CLOVES   *Caryophyllus aromaticus; Myrtaceae*

(S) *Lavanga*

(C) Ding xiang

Part Used: dried flower buds
Energetics: pungent/heating/pungent
          KV– P+
Tissues: plasma, muscle, marrow and nerve, reproductive
Actions: stimulant, expectorant, carminative, analgesic, aphrodisiac
Indications: colds, cough, asthma, indigestion, toothache, vomiting,
hiccough, laryngitis, pharyngitis, low blood pressure, impotence
Precautions: inflammatory condition, hypertension, high *Pitta*
Preparation: infusion (do not boil), powder (250 to 500 mg), milk
decoction

CLOVES are an effective stimulant and aromatic for the lungs and stomach. They dispel chill and disinfect the lymphatics. Along with rock candy, they are effective in colds and cough. The volatile oil is a powerful analgesic. Cloves are mildly aphrodisiac. They are very heating and their energizing effect may be a little irritating owing to their *rajasic* quality.

COMFREY   *Symphytum officinale; Boraginaceae*

Part Used: root and leaves
Energetics: sweet, astringent/cooling/sweet
       PV– K+
Tissues: plasma, blood, muscle, bone, marrow and nerve
Systems: respiratory, digestive, circulatory, nervous
Actions: nutritive tonic, demulcent, expectorant, emollient, vulnerary, astringent, hemostatic
Indications: cough, lung infections, coughing blood, lung hemorrhage, gastrointestinal ulcers, blood in urine, diarrhea, dysentery, sprains, fractures, wounds, sores, boils
Precautions: edema, malabsorption, obesity, high *Ama*
Preparation: decoction, milk decoction, powder (250 mg to 1 g), paste

COMFREY is a powerful tonic and vulnerary; the root has stronger tonic properties, while the leaves are more astringent and anti-inflammatory. Comfrey root is a nutritive and rejuvenative tonic to the lungs and the mucous membranes. It can be used in most conditions where membranes are inflamed, bleeding or wasting away. Comfrey is one of the best agents for promoting tissue growth, externally and internally, and healing throughout the body, when it has been afflicted by disease or traumatic injuries.

As a tonic and hemostatic, two teaspoons of powder can be boiled in one cup of milk. For expectorant action it should be combined with hot spices like ginger, cloves and cardamom as by itself it can cause congestion. As a lung tonic it can be used with elecampane root. It is a *rasayana* for *Vata* and *Pitta*, for the lungs, the plasma (*rasa dhatu*) and the bones. It is one of the most powerful agents—a true tonic—for promoting new tissue growth.

CORIANDER   *Coriandrum sativum; Umbelliferae*

(S) *Dhanyaka*

(C) Yan shi

Part Used: fruit, fresh plant (cilantro, Chinese parsley)
Energetics: Bitter, pungent/cooling/pungent
          PKV=
Tissues: plasma, blood, muscle
Systems: digestive, respiratory, urinary
Actions: alterative, diaphoretic, diuretic, carminative, stimulant
Indications: burning urethra, cystitis, urinary tract infection, urticaria, rash, burns, sore throat, vomiting, indigestion, allergies, hay fever
Precautions: few, except high *Vata* with nerve tissue deficiency
Preparation: infusion (cold or hot), powder (250 to 500 mg), fresh juice (of cilantro)

CORIANDER seeds are a good household remedy for many *Pitta* disorders, particularly those of the digestive tract or urinary system. It is an effective digestive agent for *Pitta* conditions in which most spices are contraindicated or used with caution. The fresh juice of the herb is effective internally for allergies, hay fever and skin rashes; one teaspoon three times a day, but it can also be used externally for itch and inflammation.

Similar in properties is cumin, which is an antidote for hot, pungent food (tomatoes, chilis, etc.). It increases digestion and absorption, and is good for diarrhea and dysentery. Coriander, cumin and fennel seeds are related plants with similar properties. The three are often used together for digestive disorders, mainly owing to high *Pitta*, and are used together in various formulations to promote the assimilation of the other herbs.

DANDELION   *Taraxacum officinale; Compositae*

(C) Pu gong ying

Part Used: root, herb
Energetics: bitter, sweet/cooling/pungent
          PK– V+

Tissues: plasma, blood
Systems: circulatory, digestive, urinary, lymphatic
Actions: Alterative, diuretic, lithotriptic, laxative, bitter tonic
Indications: liver problems, jaundice, gall stones, congested lymphatics, breast sores, breast cancer, hepatitis, diabetes, edema, ulcers
Precautions: high *Vata*
Preparation: decoction (root), powder (250 mg to 1 g), paste

DANDELION is primarily a detoxifying herb for *Pitta* and *Ama* conditions. It is a specific for problems of the breast and mammary glands, breast sores, tumors, cysts, suppression of lactation, swollen lymph glands. It clears and cleanses the liver and gall bladder and dispels accumulated and stagnated *Pitta* and bile.

Dandelion root combines well with chicory root or burdock root, as an anti-*Pitta* beverage (1/4 ounce of each can be simmered in one pint of water for twenty minutes and taken three times a day with meals. It is similar in properties to the Indian herb *bhringaraj*, which is a stronger tonic and nervine, and may substitute for it. Dandelion is good for detoxification from a meat diet and over-eating of fatty and fried foods.

ECHINACEA   *Echinacea angustifolia; Compositae*

Part Used: root
Energetics: bitter, pungent/cooling/pungent
          PK– V+
Tissues: plasma, blood
Systems: circulatory, lymphatic, respiratory
Actions: alterative, diaphoretic, antibacterial, antiviral, antiseptic, analgesic
Indication: toxic conditions of the blood, blood poisoning, gangrene, eczema, poisonous bites or stings, venereal diseases, prostatitis, infection, wounds, abscesses
Precautions: anemia, vertigo, high *Vata*
Preparation: infusion (hot or cold), powder (250 mg to 1 g), tincture

ECHINACEA is probably the best detoxifying agent in western herbalism. It is a natural herbal antibiotic and counters the effects of most poisons in the body. It cleanses the blood and lymph systems, catalyzes the action of the white blood cells and helps arrest pus formation and tissue putrefaction. In terms of Ayurveda, it is used in destroying *Ama*.

Its usage is somewhat similar to golden seal, but whereas golden seal acts more on the g.i. tract, echinacea is stronger on the blood and the lungs, for colds, flus, etc. Echinacea is less depleting on the body than golden seal, and so is preferable for more long term usage.

For lung infections, it combines well with its relative, elecampane. Where it may cause dizziness or ungroundedness, it can be combined with licorice or marshmallow. Unlike golden seal, echinacea can be used in normal dosages, but care must be taken to get the plant fairly fresh (it loses its potency in six months or less), which is why a tincture is often preferable.

It can be used externally as a poultice or wash for toxic bites or infectious sores.

ELECAMPANE   *Inula spp.; Compositae*

(S) *Pushkaramula*

(C) Xuan fu

Part Used: roots and flowers
Energetics: pungent, bitter/heating/pungent
          KV– P+
Tissues: all except reproductive
Systems: respiratory, nervous, digestive
Actions: expectorant, antispasmodic, carminative, analgesic, rejuvenative
Indications: colds, asthma, cardiac asthma, pleurisy, dyspepsia, cough, nervous debility
Precautions: high *Pitta* conditions generally
Preparation: decoction, powder (250 mg to 1 g), paste

ELECAMPANE is one of the best rejuvenative tonics for the lungs. It is effective for reducing excess *Kapha* and strengthening the muscles of the lungs, promoting longevity of the lung tissues. It helps to absorb water from the lungs and reduce swelling. It is one of the best expectorants and cough-relievers and has a calming action on the digestive system, the mind, and the female reproductive organs.

As a diaphoretic and expectorant it can be taken with such herbs as ginger, *pippali*, cinnamon and cardamom. As a tonic and rejuvenative it can be taken with such herbs as *ashwagandha*, comfrey root or marshmallow. It may be used externally as a paste for muscular pain, onehalf ounce may be simmered in one pint of water for 20 minutes and taken three times a day after meals, with honey, as a lung tonic.

FENNEL SEEDS   *Foeniculum vulgaris; Umbelliferae*

(S) *Shatapushpa*, what possesses a hundred flowers

(C) Xiao hue xiang

Part Used: fruit (seeds)
Energetics: sweet, pungent/cooling (slightly)/sweet
           VPK=
Tissues: plasma, blood, muscles, marrow
Systems: digestive, nervous, urinary
Actions: carminative, stomachic, stimulant, diuretic, antispasmodic
Indications: indigestion, low agni, abdominal pain, cramps or gas, difficult or burning urination, children's colic
Precautions: a good general herb and spice for all constitutions
Preparation: infusion, powder (250 to 500 mg)

FENNEL SEEDS are one of the best herbs for digestion, strengthening *Agni* without aggravating *Pitta*, stopping cramping and dispelling flatulence. They can be taken roasted after meals, one teaspoon, by themselves or with rock salt. They combine well with cumin and coriander as three cooling spices. Fennel seeds are excellent for digestive weakness in children or in the elderly. They are calming to the nerves, their aroma acts upon the mind and promotes mental alertness. For urinary problems, they combine well with coriander. Fennel can be used for digestive weakness where hot spices and peppers might overheat or overstimulate.

They work to stop the griping of purgatives and can also help promote menstruation and to promote milk flow for nursing mothers.

FENUGREEK   *Trigonella foenumgraeceum; Leguminosae*

(S) *Methi*

(C) Hu lu ba

Part Used: seeds
Energetics: bitter, pungent, sweet/heating/pungent
          VK– P+
Tissues: plasma, blood, marrow and nerve, reproductive
Systems: digestive, respiratory, urinary, reproductive
Actions: stimulant, tonic, expectorant, rejuvenative, aphrodisiac, diuretic
Indications: dysentery, dyspepsia, chronic cough, allergies, bronchitis, influenza, convalescence, dropsy, toothache, neurasthenia, sciatica, arthritis
Precautions: pregnancy (may cause abortion, promotes vaginal bleeding), high *Pitta* conditions
Preparation: decoction, powder (250 mg to 1 g), paste, gruel

FENUGREEK is a good herbal food for convalescence and debility, particularly that of the nervous, respiratory and reproductive systems. As a gruel it will increase milk flow and promote hair growth. The seed paste can be used externally for boils, ulcers and hard to heal sores. With valerian it is a good nerve tonic. It can be added to curries as a digestion-promoting spice. Fenugreek sprouts are a medicinal vegetable for indigestion, hypo-function of the liver and seminal debility. As a tonic, one tablespoon of the powder can be taken daily, heated in one cup of milk.

FLAXSEED   *Linum usitatissimum; Linaceae*

(S) *Uma*

Part Used: seed
Energetics: sweet, astringent,/heating/pungent
      V– PK+
Tissues: plasma, blood, muscle, bone
Systems: excretory, respiratory
Actions: laxative, demulcent, emollient, expectorant, nutritive tonic
Indications: asthma, chronic bronchitis, pneumonia, chronic constipation, diarrhea, convalescence
Precautions: may not be strong enough for severe constipation and may feed congestion in the colon
Preparation: infusion, decoction, milk decoction, paste, powder (250 mg to 1 g)

FLAXSEEDS are a good tonic for *Vata*, for the colon and the lungs. They strengthen lung tissue and promote the healing of the lung membranes. They are excellent for chronic, degenerative lung disorders. They contain natural protein and calcium. As an expectorant and emollient, they combine well with honey. As a lung tonic they work well with licorice. They have similar properties to sesame seeds, particularly for strengthening the bones and the reproductive organs. As a laxative, they differ from psyllium in being lighter and hotter, better for *Vata*, generally speaking, but more likely to aggravate *Pitta*. Take a warm infusion, one teaspoon to two tablespoons per cup (depending upon strength needed) before sleep for constipation.

Externally, they make a good poultice for ulcerated and inflamed surfaces, as they help dilate local blood vessels and relax the tissue.

GARLIC   *Allium sativum; Liliaceae*

(S) *Rashona*, "lacking one taste," as it contains all of the six tastes except sour. (Pungent resides in its root, bitter in its leaf, astringent in its stem, saline at the top of the stem and sweet taste in the seed.)

(C) Da suan

Part Used: rhizome
Energetics: all but sour, mainly pungent/heating/pungent
        VK– P+
Tissues: works on all tissue-elements
Systems: digestive, respiratory, nervous, reproductive, circulatory
Actions: stimulant, carminative, expectorant, alterative, antispasmodic, aphrodisiac, disinfectant, anthelmintic, rejuvenative
Indications: colds, cough, asthma, heart disease, hypertension, cholesterol, arteriosclerosis, palpitation, skin diseases, parasitic infections, rheumatism, hemorrhoids, edema, impotence, hysteria
Precautions: hyperacidity, toxic heat in the blood, high *Pitta*
Preparation: infusion (do not boil), powder (100 to 500 mg), juice, medicated oil

GARLIC is a powerful rejuvenative herb. It is a *rasayana* for *Vata*, and also, to a lesser degree, for *Kapha*, for the bone and nerve tissue. It also is a powerful detoxifier and is good for chronic or periodic (*Vata*) fevers. It cleanses *Ama* and *Kapha* from the blood and lymphatics. Yet its heating attribute can aggravate the blood and cause or aggravate bleeding.

Its quality is *tamasic*. Garlic can increase dullness of mind while, on the other hand, may increase "groundedness." It increases semen but also has an irritant effect upon the reproductive organs. So while good as a medicine, garlic may not be a good common-usage herb for those practicing yoga.

GENTIAN   *Gentiana spp.; Gentianaceae*

(S) *Kirata, Katuki, Trayamana* (several bitter herbs are used almost as equivalents and so the nomenclature is not entirely specific)

(C) Long dan cao

Part Used: root
Energetics: bitter/cooling/pungent
        PK– V+
Tissues: plasma, blood, muscle, fat
Systems: circulatory, digestive
Actions: bitter tonic, antipyretic, alterative, antibacterial, anthelmintic, laxative

Indications: fever, debility after fevers, jaundice, hepatitis, enlargement of liver and spleen, genital herpes, acne, rash, obesity, ulcers, venereal sores, diabetes, cancer
Precautions: general debility, nervousness, muscle spasms, high *Vata*
Preparation: decoction, powder (250 to 500 mg)

GENTIAN is a classic bitter herb of world-wide usage, a typical bitter tonic. Like most bitter herbs, it destroys *Ama* in fever and inflammation. It is a strong herb for sedating hyperactivity of the liver and spleen, and it heals genital area sores and infections. It is good for ulcers in the stomach and small intestine. It is one of the best anti-*Pitta* herbs.

For reducing fever it may be given with equal amounts of dry ginger or black pepper. For regulating liver-spleen function it combines well with aloe vera and may be taken along with aloe as an *anupana*.

However, where there is no fever or inflammation, or where there is no high *Pitta* or excess fat in the body, it is not to be used. *Vata*-type nervous digestion and hypoglycemia will not respond well to it.

It has value in such modern diseases as genital herpes and cancer, particularly diseases of a *Pitta* nature, or those rooted in the blood or liver.

GINGER   *Zingiber officinale; Zingiberaceae*

(S) *Sunthi, Nagara* (dry), *Ardraka* (fresh)

(C) Gan jiang (dry), Shen jiang (fresh)

Part Used: rhizome
Energetics: pungent, sweet/heating/sweet
       VK– P+
Tissues: works on all tissue-elements
Systems: digestive, respiratory
Actions: stimulant, diaphoretic, expectorant, carminative, antiemetic, analgesic
Indications: colds, flus, indigestion, vomiting, belching, abdominal pain, laryngitis, arthritis, hemorrhoids, headaches, heart disease
Precautions: inflammatory skin diseases, high fever, bleeding, ulcers
Preparation: infusion, decoction, powder (250 to 500 mg), fresh juice

GINGER is perhaps the best and most *sattvic* of the spices. It was called *vishwabhesaj*, "the universal medicine." As such, it was prepared by adding fresh ginger juice to ginger powder, mixing it in a mortar and pestle, until it became a thick jam, whereupon it was rolled into pills. The proportion of juice to powder was upwards of 4 to 1. Two pills, about the size of a pea, were taken three times a day. With honey, ginger relieves *Kapha*; with rock candy it relieves *Pitta*; with rock salt it relieves *Vata*.

Dry ginger is hotter and drier than fresh. It is a better stimulant and expectorant for reducing *Kapha* and increasing *Agni*. Fresh ginger is a better diaphoretic, better for colds, cough, vomiting and for deranged *Vata*.

The uses of ginger in digestive and respiratory diseases are well known. It is also good in arthritic conditions and it is tonic to the heart. It relieves gas and cramps in the abdomen, including menstrual cramps due to cold. Externally, it makes a good paste for pain and headaches.

GOLDEN SEAL   *Hydrastis canadensis; Ranunculaceae*

Part Used: rhizome
Energetics: Bitter, astringent/cooling/pungent
           PK– V+
Tissues: plasma, blood
Systems: digestive, circulatory, lymphatic
Actions: bitter tonic, antipyretic, alterative, antibiotic, antibacterial, antiseptic, laxative
Indications: jaundice, hepatitis, diabetes, obesity, ulcers, infectious fever, malaria, swollen glands and lymphatics, hemorrhoids, eczema, pyorrhea, menorrhagia, leucorrhea
Precautions: emaciation, neurasthenia, vertigo, chronic debility, (prolonged usage should be less than 3 gms. per day)
Preparation: decoction, powder (100 to 500 mg), paste (externally)

GOLDEN SEAL is a good herbal antibiotic, antibacterial and antiseptic agent. It destroys yeast and bacteria in the gastrointestinal tract and clears the flora. Its strong detoxifying action extends throughout the circulatory system as well. It sedates and regulates liver and spleen function, along with sugar and fat metabolism, reducing toxins and excess tissue from the body. It purifies the mucous membranes and is good for all catarrhal conditions.

However, it is not a panacea for all diseases. It has a negative impact on good intestinal flora and has many of the contraindications of antibiotic drugs (it is good to use in place of them). It is contraindicated in most deficiency conditions, most conditions where a nurturing therapy is appropriate.

For deep-seated fevers it can be combined with hot herbs like ginger or black pepper. As an astringent gargle or mouthwash it can be used with myrrh.

It is perhaps the strongest anti-*Pitta* herb available in this country.

HAWTHORN BERRIES   *Crataegus oxycantha; Rosaceae*

(C) Shan sha

Part Used: fruit
Energetics: sour/heating/sour
         V– P+ K+ (in excess)
Tissues: plasma, blood, muscles
Systems: circulatory, digestive
Actions: stimulant, carminative, vasodilator, antispasmodic, diuretic
Indications: heart weakness, arteriosclerosis, valvular insufficiency, hypertension, palpitations, blood clots, insomnia, food stagnation, abdominal tumors
Precautions: ulcers, colitis
Preparation: decoction, powder (250 mg to 1 g)

HAWTHORN BERRIES are a good example of the stimulatory power of sour herbs for both circulation and digestion. They have a special action on the heart, strengthening the heart muscle and promoting longevity. They are particularly good for *Vata* heart conditions like nervous palpitation, or the heart problems of old age (the age of *Vata*) like cholesterol and arteriosclerosis.

In promoting digestion they help remove accumulated food masses or even tumors in the gastrointestinal tract. Yet they can help increase weight in the body and may aggravate *Kapha* in excess. They will also aggravate most *Pitta* heart conditions and heat conditions in the body generally.

They can be prepared as a tincture or herbal wine—they have an affinity for alcohol. For strengthening the heart muscles, they can be used with other heart tonics like small amounts of cardamom and cinnamon. One-half ounce of hawthorn berries can be simmered in one pint of water for 20 minutes along with one teaspoon of cinnamon and taken three times a day after meals, sweetened with honey as a heart tonic.

HIBISCUS FLOWERS   *Hibiscus rosa-sinensis; Malvaceae*

(S) *Japa*, strengthens devotion in japa, repetition of the *mantra*

Part Used: flowers
Energetics: astringent, sweet/cooling/sweet
                  PK– V+ (in excess)
Tissues: blood, plasma, muscles, marrow and nerve, reproductive
Systems: circulatory, female reproductive, nervous
Actions: alterative, hemostatic, refrigerant, emmenagogue, demulcent, antispasmodic
Indications: dysmennorhea, menorrhagia, painful urination, cystitis, cough, fever, venereal diseases, toxins in blood
Precautions: severe chills, high *Vata*
Preparation: infusion (cold or hot), powder (250 mg to 1 g)

HIBISCUS FLOWERS are good for first and second *chakra* disorders, such as problems of the kidneys and reproductive systems due to heat, congestion and contraction. They make a good summer beverage to reduce heat and fever; 1/4 ounce of the flowers let set in one pint cool water.

Hibiscus flowers are sacred to *Ganesh*, the elephant god, the god of wisdom who destroys all obstacles and grants the realization of all goals, who dwells in the first or root *chakra*. They help make *mantras* fruitful, give *siddhis* (occult powers) and enhance attention in meditation. They are an important part of all *pujas* (devotional ceremonies) and have a similar energy to lotus flowers and rose flowers, the last of which they combine well with for most purposes.

Hibiscus flowers help purify the blood and the heart, physically and spiritually, and they also improve skin complexion and promote hair growth. They are effective in menstrual difficulties, particularly excessive bleeding.

HORSETAIL   *Equisetum spp.; Equisetaceae*

(C) Mu zei

Part Used: herb
Energetics: bitter, sweet/cooling/pungent
      PK– V+
Tissues: plasma, blood, fat, bone
Systems: urinary, respiratory
Actions: diuretic, lithotriptic, diaphoretic, alterative, hemostatic
Indications: edema, nephritis, burning urethra, kidney stones, gall bladder stones, stomach ulcers, broken bones, menorrhagia, venereal diseases
Precaution: high *Vata*, constipation, dry skin
Preparation: infusion (hot or cold), powder (250 to 500 mg), paste

HORSETAIL is an effective diuretic and blood cleanser. It is a good general herb for high *Pitta* conditions and has a strong stone-removing action for kidney, bladder and gall-stones. Yet it is somewhat of an irritant and an abrasive in its action and should not be taken for long periods of time without proper supervision. Horsetail promotes the healing of broken bones and supplies nutrients to the bone tissue. It helps clear and brighten the eyes and removes toxicity from the blood. It is also good for infectious fevers and flus.

Horsetail has similar properties to burdock seeds and can be used externally as a paste or wash for inflamed surfaces. It clears *Pitta* and fiery emotions from the nerves and mind.

IRISH MOSS   *Chondrus crispus; Algae*

Part Used: herb
Energetics: salty, sweet, astringent/heating (slightly)/sweet
          VP– K or *Ama* + (in excess)
Tissues: plasma, muscle, fat
Systems: respiratory, urinary
Actions: nutritive tonic, demulcent, expectorant, emollient
Indications: cough, bronchitis, tuberculosis, enlarged glands (thyroid, lymph, prostate), convalescence, debility, old age, dry or wrinkled skin
Precautions: high *Ama*, congestion
Preparation: infusion, decoction, milk decoction, powder (250 mg to 1 g), paste

IRISH MOSS and other forms of seaweed, like kelp or dulse, are good herbal foods for deficient conditions, convalescence, old age, high *Vata* and hormonal, particularly thyroid, insufficiency. They are restoratives and rejuvenatives to *rasa*, the basic plasma tissue-element of the body, increasing our basic fluids and enriching them with minerals. They soften and help remove dried out *Kapha* and *Ama* accumulations in the lungs. By soothing and nurturing the glands, they help reduce swelling. They are effective (internally and externally) for soothing dried and inflamed surfaces or membranes.

One-half ounce of Irish moss may be simmered in one pint of water and taken in two parts daily for convalescence from severe lung diseases.

JUNIPER BERRIES   *Juniperus spp.; Coniferae*

(S) *Hapusha*

Part Used: berries
Energetics: pungent, bitter, sweet/heating/pungent
          KV– P+
Tissues: plasma, blood, muscle, fat, bone, marrow and nerves
Systems: urinary, respiratory, nervous, digestive
Actions: diuretic, diaphoretic, stimulant, carminative, analgesic, disinfectant, bacteriocidal

Indications: dropsy, edema, sciatica, lumbago, arthritis, rheumatism, swollen joints, diabetes, weak digestion, weak immune system, dysmenorrhea
Precautions: acute nephritis, cystitis, pregnancy
Preparation: infusion, powder (250 to 500 mg), paste

JUNIPER BERRIES are one of the best diuretics for *Vata* constitution, as they also dispel excess *Vata* and improve digestion. They are also very good for *Kapha* but will aggravate *Pitta*, and so must be used with other diuretics with proper consideration. They are often given with demulcent diuretics, like marshmallow or *gokshura*, to balance out their irritant properties. As a paste they may be applied externally for arthritic pain and swelling. Their purifying action extends to the aura and the subtle body, as they help destroy not only resistant bacteria but also negative astral influences.

LICORICE   *Glycyrrhiza glabra; Leguminosae*

(S) *Yashti Madhu*, honey-stick

(C) Gan cao

Part Used: root
Energetics: sweet, bitter/cooling/sweet
       VP– K+ (if used long term)
Tissues: works on all tissue-elements
Systems: digestive, respiratory, nervous, reproductive, excretory
Actions: demulcent, expectorant, tonic, rejuvenative, laxative, sedative, emetic
Indications: cough, colds, bronchitis, sore throat, laryngitis, ulcers, hyperacidity, painful urination, abdominal pain, general debility
Precautions: high *Kapha*, edema; inhibits absorption of calcium and potassium, not for osteoporosis; hypertension (increases water around the heart)
Preparation: decoction, milk decoction, powder (250 to 500 mg), medicated *ghee*

LICORICE is an effective expectorant, helping to liquify mucus and facilitate its discharge from the body. In large doses it is a good emetic for cleansing the lungs and stomach of *Kapha*. It is a mild laxative which soothes and tones the mucous membranes, relieving muscle spasms and reducing inflammation. Its taste masks the disagreeable flavor of other herbs and helps harmonize their qualities, countering heat and dryness and reducing toxicity.

For colds and respiratory affliction, it combines well with fresh ginger. With ginger and cardamom it is a tonic to the teeth. It is a restorative and rejuvenative food. *Sattvic* in quality, it calms the mind and nurtures the spirit. It nourishes the brain and increases cranial and cerebrospinal fluid, promoting contentment and harmony. It improves voice, vision, hair and complexion and gives strength.

MARSHMALLOW   *Althea officinalis; Malvaceae*

Part Used: root
Energetics: sweet/cooling/sweet
          VPK= (may increase *Kapha* or *Ama* in excess)
Tissues: plasma, blood, muscle, marrow and nerve, reproductive
Systems: respiratory, urinary, digestive, nervous
Actions: nutritive tonic, rejuvenative, demulcent, expectorant, emollient, diuretic, vulnerary, laxative
Indications: cough, whooping cough, laryngitis, bronchitis, kidney and bladder inflammation, infection or bleeding, skin eruptions, mastitis, malnutrition, burns, rheumatism
Precautions: malabsorption
Preparation: decoction, milk decoction, powder (250 mg to 1 g), paste

MARSHMALLOW contains large amounts of high quality mucilage and is perhaps the best nutritive tonic herb (internally) and softening emollient (externally) in western herbalism. It is rejuvenative for *Pitta*, for the lungs and the kidneys and also tonifies *Vata*. It allays inflammation, soothes the skin and the mucous membranes and simultaneously cleanses and rebuilds the water element in the body. It promotes the healing of chronic sores and necrotic tissue.

Because it has a strong drawing property, it can be used externally as a poultice for inflammations and infections. As a rejuvenative it can be decocted in milk and a small amount of ginger. As a lung tonic, it combines well with licorice and elecampane root. It is a good soothing and harmonizing herb for any diuretic formula; for allaying cough it works well with thyme.

The wild mallows can be used in a similar fashion, though large roots are required for the strongest tonic action. For Indian relatives and herbs of similar usage see *bala*.

MINT   *Mentha spp.; Labiatae*

(S) *Phudina*

(C) Ba he

Part Used: herb
Energetics: pungent/cooling (slightly)/pungent
            PK– V+ (in excess)
Tissues: plasma, blood, marrow and nerves
Systems: respiratory, digestive, nervous, circulatory
Actions: stimulant, diaphoretic, carminative, nervine, analgesic
Indications: colds, fever, sore throat, laryngitis, earache, digestive upset, nervous agitation, headache, dysmenorrhea
Precautions: severe chills, neurasthenia
Preparation: infusion (do not boil), powder (250 to 500 mg)

The three main mints, PEPPERMINT, SPEARMINT and HORSE-MINT (Mentha arvensis, which is more common in India and also a wild mint native to the western United States) have a mild soothing action on the nerves and digestion, which helps relax the body and clear the mind and senses, hence their widespread popularity and usage. They are mild, cooling diaphoretics for common colds and flus and their complications. Peppermint is the most stimulating and the best one to improve digestion. Spearmint is more relaxing and better in diuretic action (i.e. for urinary inflammation). Horsemint has stronger antispasmodic properties, as for difficult menstruation. Other mints like catnip have similar properties, but not all mints are cooling. Some, like thyme, are heating. But most are not excessively heating or cooling.

Mints contain large amounts of the element of ether, whose action is soothing, cooling, clarifying and expanding. Through their ethereal nature they help relieve mental and emotional tension and congestion. Their nature is *sattvic*. Their action on the body is mild and not strong enough for acute or severe ailments. They are usually used with other herbs in an auxiliary role as harmonizing agents or as *anupanas*.

MUGWORT   *Artemesia vulgaris; Compositae*

(S) *Nagadamani*

(C) Ai ye

Part Used: herb
Energetics: bitter, pungent/heating/pungent
             VK– P+ (in excess)
Tissues: skin, blood, muscles, marrow and nerve
Systems: circulatory, female reproductive, nervous, digestive, respiratory
Actions: emmenagogue, antispasmodic, hemostatic, diaphoretic, anthelmintic, antiseptic
Indications: dysmenorrhea, menorrhagia, infertility, preventive for miscarriage, sciatica, convulsions, hysteria, epilepsy, depression, mental exhaustion, insomnia, gout, rheumatism, fungal infections
Precautions: high *Pitta*, uterine infection or inflammation
Preparation: infusion (do not overboil), powder (250 to 500 mg)

Various members of the Artemesia species are used medicinally throughout the world, including mugwort, wormwood, southernwood, and the sagebrush of the Great Basin region. All possess similar properties as bitter aromatics. Of these, mugwort is the better emmenagogue; wormwood is better for killing worms and strengthening digestion; and sagebrush appears to be a better diaphoretic. They are particularly good for *sama Vata* conditions, such as arthritis or for nervous conditions owing to obstructed *Vata*.

MUGWORT warms the lower abdomen and fortifies the uterus. It regulates menstruation, relieves menstrual cramping and headaches, and strengthens the fetus. It opens and purifies the channels (the cir-

culatory and nervous system), and relieves pain. It can be used with
ginger and pennyroyal to promote menstruation blocked by nervous
tension. Externally it can be used as a wash for fungal and other skin
infections, or as a douch (infusion) for vaginal yeast infections.

MULLEIN   *Verbascum thapsus; Scrophulariaceae*

Part Used: herb, flowers
Energetics: bitter, astringent, sweet/cooling/pungent
          PK– V+
Tissues: plasma, blood, marrow and nerve
Systems: respiratory, nervous, circulatory, lymphatic
Actions: expectorant, astringent, vulnerary, antispasmodic, analgesic,
sedative
Indications: bronchitis, asthma, hay fever, dyspnea, sinusitis, cough,
lung hemorrhage, swollen glands, earache, mumps, nerve pain, insom-
nia, diarrhea, dysentery
Precautions: high *Vata*
Preparation: infusion (hot or cold—strain well), powder (250 to
500 mg), oil (flowers)

MULLEIN is a powerful herb for dispelling heat and congestion from
the lungs and nasal passages. It dispels accumulated *Kapha*, cleansing
the bronchii and the lymphatics. It is specific for mumps, earaches and
glandular swellings. The flowers have stronger nervine and analgesic
properties, with the flower oil being a powerful and anti-
inflammatory anodyne. Mullein flowers relieve inflammation of the
nerve tissue, and allay irritation.

An ounce of mullein leaves can be decocted in a pint of milk and
taken before sleep, one cup, to relieve cough and promote sleep that
has been disturbed by cough and congestion.

MYRRH   *Commiphora myrrha; Burseraceae*

(S) *Bola*

(C) Mu yao

Part Used: Resin

Energetics: bitter, astringent, pungent, sweet/heating/pungent
         KV– P+ (in excess)
Tissues: works on all tissue-elements
Systems: circulatory, reproductive, nervous, lymphatic, respiratory
Actions: alterative, emmenagogue, astringent, expectorant, antispas-
modic, rejuvenative, analgesic, antiseptic
Indications: amenorrhea, dysmenorrhea, menopause, cough, asthma,
bronchitis, arthritis, rheumatism, traumatic injuries, ulcerated surfaces,
anemia, pyorrhea
Precautions: high *Pitta*
Preparation: infusion, powder (250 mg to 1 g), pill, paste

MYRRH is one of the most famous and ancient substances used for
preventing decay, reversing the aging process and rejuvenating body
and mind. It is closely related to the *guggul* of Ayurvedic medicine, an
important Ayurvedic *rasayana*. Myrrh similarly is a rejuvenative for
Vata and *Kapha*, but it works more specifically on the blood and the
female reproductive system; *guggul* possesses a stronger action on the
nerves. Myrrh helps dispel old and stagnant blood from the uterus,
and aids in new tissue growth. It catalyzes healing of sores and
wounds, while stopping pain. It also helps dispel repressed emotions,
as its purifying action extends to the subtle body.

Myrrh possesses true tonic, stimulant and rejuvenative powers along
with strong detoxifying effects. As such, it is a more powerful and
balanced herb than golden seal and other bitter detoxifiers, which
weaken the body in long term usage. Yet it is not as effective as these
in acute conditions.

Frankincense or Olibanum, Boswellia carterii, has very similar properties also, but has a slightly stronger action on the lungs and the nervous system.

As a general tonic for *Vata* or *Kapha* or for the female reproductive system, two '00' capsules of myrrh can be taken three times a day.

NUTMEG
Myristica fragrans; Myristicaceae

(S) *Jatiphala*

(C) Rou dou kou

Part Used: fruit (seed)
Energetics: pungent/heating/pungent
       VK– P+
Tissues: plasma, muscle, marrow and nerve, reproductive
Systems: digestive, nervous, reproductive
Actions: astringent, carminative, sedative, nervine, aphrodisiac, stimulant
Indications: poor absorption, abdominal pain and distension, diarrhea, dysentery, intestinal gas, insomnia, nervous disorders, impotence
Precautions: pregnancy, high *Pitta*
Preparation: infusion (do not boil), milk decoction, powder (250 to 500 mg)

NUTMEG is one of the best spices for increasing absorption, particularly in the small intestine. It works well in this respect with such spices as cardamom and ginger. Taken in buttermilk, it improves assimilation and stops diarrhea. It helps reduce high *Vata* in the colon and in the nervous system. It is one of the best medicines for calming the mind. For this it can be taken 500 mg. in warm milk before sleep, to promote sound sleep. However, it has a *tamasic* quality, somewhat like poppy seeds, and in excess can increase dullness of mind.

It is good for incontinence of urine or for premature ejaculation. It also serves to relieve muscle-spasms, particularly of the abdomen.

PARSLEY
Petroselinum spp.; Umbelliferae

Part Used: herb, root, seeds
Energetics: pungent, bitter (herb); sweet, bitter (root)/heating
       (slightly)/pungent
       KV– P+ (in excess)
Tissues: plasma, blood, muscles
Systems: urinary, digestive, female reproductive

Actions: diuretic, lithotriptic, emmenagogue, laxative, carminative, antispasmodic

Indications: dropsy, edema, swollen glands, swollen breasts, amenorrhea, dysmenorrhea, gall stones, kidney stones, lumbago, sciatica

Precautions: acute inflammation of kidneys or female reproductive system, high *Pitta*

Preparation: infusion (herb and seeds), decoction (root), juice (herb), powder (250 to 500 mg)

PARSLEY is rich in minerals, vitamins and iron and so is a good herbal nutritional supplement. It is also a good, mildly warming diuretic which can be used in many conditions of chill and weakness where most other diuretics would be contraindicated. It is an effective emmenagogue that promotes menstruation, relieves premenstrual cramping and headaches, and dispels premenstrual water retention from the abdomen, the legs and the breast. It also helps dispel kidney and gall stones. Yet owing to its heating energy, it should be used with care when there is much inflammation or irritation of the kidneys. For such conditions it can be balanced out by combining it with marshmallow. It is good for high *Kapha* and obstructed *Vata*.

The fresh juice (2 teaspoons) may be taken daily to strengthen the kidneys and the uterus. Parsley is similar in action to, but milder than, juniper berries.

PENNYROYAL   *Mentha pulegium; Labiatae*

Part Used: herb

Energetics: pungent/heating/pungent
                VK− P+ (in excess)

Tissues: plasma, blood, marrow and nerve

Systems: female reproductive, circulatory, nervous, respiratory

Actions: emmenagogue, stimulant, carminative, antispasmodic, anthelmintic, antivenomous

Indications: amenorrhea, menstrual cramping, hysteria, nervousness, headache, colds, fevers

Precautions: pregnancy, uterine bleeding

Preparation: infusion, powder (250 to 500 mg), medicated oil

PENNYROYAL clears the channels of the nervous and female reproductive systems. Thereby it promotes menstruation and relieves spasms, dispelling obstructive *Vata*. It warms the uterus and relaxes the uterine muscles.

It works well on delayed menstruation due to cold, exposure or shock, for which conditions it combines well with such herbs as mugwort and ginger; for example, 1/4 ounce of pennyroyal along with one teaspoon of ginger powder can be steeped in one pint of water for 20 minutes and taken before meals to promote menstruation. Its quality is *sattvic*, it clears the mind and helps transmute female sexual energy.

Externally, the oil is a good insect repellant and has antivenomous properties.

POMEGRANATE   *Punica granatum; Lythraceae*

(S) *Dadima*

Part Used: fruit rind, rootbark, fruit
Energetics: astringent, bitter (fruit rind and rootbark); sweet, sour (fruit)/cooling/sweet
  sweet variety is said to alleviate all three *doshas*, the sour variety may aggravate *Pitta*; the common pomegranate is the sweet variety and may increase *Ama*
Tissues: plasma, blood, muscle, marrow and nerve
Systems: digestive, circulatory
Actions: astringent tonic, alterative, hemostatic, anthelmintic, refrigerant, stomachic
Indications: worms (round, pin, particularly tape), sore throat, ulcers, colitis, diarrhea, dysentery, prolapse of rectum or vagina, leucorrhea, conjunctivitis, anemia, chronic bronchitis, tuberculosis
Precautions: constipation
Preparation: decoction, powder (250 to 500 mg), fresh juice, paste

The POMEGRANATE tree is an excellent pharmacy in itself. The rootbark is a strong anthelmintic, taken as a decoction with a little cloves, followed by a purgative every second or third day to dispel the worms (such treatment may continue for 10 days or more). The fruit rind is better for usage as an astringent and anti-inflammatory herb for the mucous membranes. The fresh juice has stronger tonic properties, particularly for the blood and for *Pitta*.

The fruit rind powder may be used as a douche for leucorrhea; the paste can be used externally for sores, ulcers, hemorrhoids. The juice is good for promoting digestion and all parts have stomachic properties, which can be augmented with small amounts of cinnamon and cloves.

POPPY SEEDS   *Papaver spp.; Papaveraceae*

(S) *Ahiphena,* serpent's poison, for its narcotic properties

(C) Ying su qiao

Part used: seeds (non-narcotic)
Energetics: pungent, astringent, sweet/heating/sweet
          VK– P+
Tissues: plasma, blood, muscle, bone, marrow and nerves
Systems: nervous, digestive, respiratory, circulatory
Actions: astringent, carminative, antispasmodic, sedative, analgesic
Indications: diarrhea, dysentery, children's diarrhea, abdominal pain, poor absorption, cough, insomnia, nerve pain
Precautions: gastritis, colitis, high *Pitta*
Preparation: infusion, powder (250 mg to 1 g)

POPPY SEEDS are similar in properties to nutmeg and are often used in conjunction with it. They are a good astringent for the intestines, possessing carminative and stomachic properties, thus also increasing *Agni* while promoting absorption. They are effective for nervous digestive disorders of children or of high *Vata* types. They strengthen the villi of the small intestine. As a spice, they are antidotal to the gas-producing properties of legumes.

Their quality is *tamasic.* They induce sleep and, in long term usage, dull the mind and so may inhibit awareness, though they do help bring down high *Vata* psychological imbalances. As a nervine they may be used with valerian.

One-quarter ounce of poppy seeds can be simmered in one pint of water along with one teaspoon each of nutmeg and ginger powder and taken three times a day immediately after meals for nervous digestion. A cup may also be taken before sleep to promote rest.

PRICKLY ASH *Xanthoxylum spp.; Rutaceae*

(S) *Tumburu*

(C) Hua jiao

Part Used: seed, bark
Energetics: pungent, bitter/heating/pungent
      VK– P+
Tissues: plasma, blood, muscles
Systems: digestive, circulatory
Actions: stimulant, carminative, alterative, antiseptic, anthelmintic, analgesic
Indications: weak digestion, cold abdominal pain, chronic chill, lumbago, chronic arthritis and rheumatism, skin diseases, worms, yeast infections
Precautions: high *Pitta*, acute inflammatory conditions of the g.i. tract, pregnancy (may promote miscarriage)
Preparation: infusion, decoction, medicated oil, powder (250 to 500 mg), capsules

PRICKLY ASH is a powerful toxin-destroying herb (*Ama-pachana*). It destroys toxins in the g.i. tract, including worms, and is good for treating yeast infections, candida, either in the g.i. tract or in the blood. It is particularly good for *sama Vata* and arthritic conditions. It has a warming, stimulating and purifying influence on the blood and increases peripheral circulation. It relieves abdominal pain, colic and cramps.

As an antirheumatic agent, it works well with juniper berries or eucalyptus. As a digestive agent, it works well with dry ginger. For yeast infections where there is inflammation, it can be combined with bitter herbs like golden seal. For obstinate sores and chronic skin conditions, it can be used with myrrh. It can be prepared as a medicated oil in sesame oil for an antiarthritic massage oil.

PSYLLIUM   *Plantago psyllium; Plantaginaceae*

(S) *Snigdhajira*

Part Used: seeds, seed husks
Energetics: sweet, astringent/cooling/sweet
      PV– K and *Ama*+
Tissues: plasma, blood
Systems: excretory, digestive
Actions: laxative, demulcent, emollient, astringent, expectorant
Indications: chronic constipation, chronic diarrhea and dysentery,
colitis, catarrh, urethritis, cystitis, gastritis, ulcers
Precautions: may create congestion and food stagnation in
the g.i. tract
Preparation: infusion, powder (500 mg to 2 g), paste

PSYLLIUM SEEDS are perhaps the best lubricating, bulk laxative
(take 1 teaspoon to 1/2 ounce of seeds, depending upon the severity of
the condition, in water. Do not steep). The seeds swell with mucilage
in the colon, which absorbs bacteria and toxins, soothes inflamed
mucous membranes and moistens dryness. Psyllium seeds, however,
may cause griping. They may be replaced with psyllium husks, which
are a superior medicinal, or balanced by an aromatic like ginger or fennel. The heavy property of psyllium tends to reduce *Agni,* and so for
long term usage balancing it out with a digestive stimulant would be
recommended anyway.

Psyllium can be taken in buttermilk in case of diarrhea, and in warm
milk in case of constipation. The powder can be used externally as a
poultice for skin irritation; for rheumatic pain for its soothing action.

RASPBERRY   *Rubus spp.; Rosaceae*

Part Used: leaves
Energetics: astringent, sweet/cooling/sweet
      PK– V+ (in excess)
Tissues: blood, plasma, muscles, reproductive
Systems: circulatory, female reproductive, digestive
Actions: astringent, alterative, tonic, hemostatic, antiemetic

Indications: diarrhea, dysentery, intestinal flu, vomiting, dysmenorrhea, menorrhagia, uterine bleeding, prolapse of uterus or anus,
hemorrhoids, inflamed mucous membranes, sores, wounds
Precautions: American red raspberry has a good reputation for reducing miscarriage but other varieties are known to promote abortion;
high *Vata*; chronic constipation
Preparation: infusion (cold or hot), powder (250 mg to 1 g), paste

RASPBERRY is an effective anti-*Pitta* herb with affinity to the colon
and female reproductive organs, where it has a strongly astringent and
mildly tonifying (nurturing) action. It raises prolapse, stops hemorrhage, gives tone to the muscles of the lower abdomen, soothes the
mucous membranes and allays inflammation. It is a safe, mild astringent for sore throats, diarrhea (it is good for children), nausea, heart-
burn and ulcers.

As a uterine tonic it can be combined with stronger tonics like
shatavari, in proportions of 1 to 3. For menstrual complaints it combines well with rose flowers and hibiscus flowers. As a good astringent douche for uterine inflammation, leucorrhea or prolapse, it can be
combined with small amounts of myrrh.

RED CLOVER   *Trifolium pratense; Leguminosae*
(S) *Vana-methika*

Part Used: flowers
Energetics: bitter, sweet/cooling/pungent
          PK– V+
Tissues: plasma, blood
Systems: circulatory, respiratory, lymphatic
Properties: alterative, diuretic, expectorant, antispasmodic
Indications: cough, bronchitis, skin eruptions, infections, cancer
Precautions: few, perhaps high *Vata*; tissue deficiency
Preparation: infusion (hot or cold), decoction, powder (250 mg to 1 g)

RED CLOVER is a mild blood purifier which is suitable for general
consumption and long term usage. Its taste is pleasant and it is mildly
strengthening. It can be used with children, the elderly or in conditions of debility, where blood purification is needed but where the

patient is weak and stronger herbal alteratives may weaken the blood. Its effectiveness in cancer is mainly in large amounts or with other antitumor agents.

Externally, it is a good wash for dry and scaly skin, and as a paste or poultice for sores that do not heal, it is particularly good.

For more acute and infectious conditions other alteratives, like echinacea or barberry, are stronger.

RHUBARB   *Rheum spp.; Polygonaceae*

(S) *Amla-vetasa*

(C) Da huang

Part Used: root
Energetics: bitter/cooling/pungent
             PK– V+
Tissues: plasma, blood, fat
Systems: excretory, digestive
Actions: purgative, alterative, hemostatic, antipyretic, anthelmintic
Indications: constipation (particularly that accompanying fevers, ulcers or infections), diarrhea and dysentery (*Pitta*-type), jaundice, liver problems, skin inflammations
Precautions: pregnancy, chronic diarrhea, chills, use with caution on hemorrhoids (not good for *Vata*-type)
Preparation: infusion, powder (1 gm as laxative, 3 gms as purgative)

RHUBARB is one of the best purgative herbs. It is stronger than flax-seeds or triphala but milder than senna. It has an astringent after-effect that protects the tone of the colon. It is good for all manner of constipation and for febrile or damp-heat diarrhea. On weaker or older patients, where there is much dryness in the colon, it can be combined with licorice and sweet, bulk laxatives, like psyllium or flax-seeds. As it tends to cause griping, it should be used with a carmina-tive herb like ginger or fennel seeds in a ratio of about 4 parts rhubarb to 1 part ginger, for example.

Rhubarb purges the body of *Pitta*, bile, *Ama*, stagnant food and stag-nant blood. It helps reduce weight and remove fat. It is mildly nauseating and so is easier taken in capsules. Rhubarb is a safe and effective remedy for children because it seldom causes irritation in the right dosage. Its action is made stronger by combining it with epsom salts.

ROSE FLOWERS   *Rosa spp.; Rosaceae*

(S) *Shatapatri*

(C) Yeu ji hua

Part Used: flowers
Energetics: bitter, pungent, astringent, sweet/cooling/sweet
               VPK= (may increase *Kapha* or *Ama* in excess)
Tissues: plasma, blood, marrow and nerve, reproductive
Systems: circulatory, female reproductive, nervous
Actions: alterative, emmenagogue, refrigerant, nervine, carminative, laxative, astringent
Indications: amenorrhea, dysmenorrhea, uterine hemorrhage, inflamed eyes, dizziness, headaches, sore throat, enlarged tonsils
Precautions: high *Kapha*
Preparation: infusion (hot or cold), powder (250 mg to 1 g), rose water

ROSE FLOWERS are particularly good for reducing *Pitta*. They relieve heat, congestion of the blood and soothe inflamed surfaces. Fresh rose petals can be macerated in honey or raw sugar and used for sore throat or mouth sores; or they may be taken with warm milk as a mild laxative for *Pitta* individuals.

Rose water can be prepared by boiling fresh petals and condensing the steam into another vessel. It opens the mind and heart and is cooling and refreshing to the eyes. Rose is a well known flower of love and devotion of *Bhakti* and of *Puja*, of devotional worship. The lotus of the heart is a rose.

As a tonic, rose flowers combine well with *shatavari*. For regulating menstruation, they combine well with safflower or hibiscus.

SAFFRON   *Crocus sativus; Iridaceae*

(S) *Nagakeshara*

Part Used: flower (stigma)
Energetics: pungent, bitter, sweet/cooling/sweet
           VPK=
Tissues: works on all tissue-elements but particularly the blood
Systems: circulatory, digestive, female reproductive, nervous
Actions: alterative, emmenagogue, aphrodisiac, rejuvenative, stimulant, carminative, antispasmodic
Indications: menstrual pain and irregularity, menopause, impotence, infertility, anemia, enlarged liver, hysteria, depression, neuralgia, lumbago, rheumatism, cough, asthma, chronic diarrhea
Precautions: pregnancy (can promote miscarriage), in large doses is narcotic
Preparation: infusion, milk decoction, powder (100 to 250 mg); use in low dosages, a pinchful with other herbs, medicated oil, medicated *ghee*

SAFFRON is a very potent but expensive revitalizer of the blood, circulation and female reproductive system, as well as of the metabolism generally. It is one of the best anti-*Pitta* herbs and spleen-liver regulators. It is considered to be the best stimulant and aphrodisiac, *vajikarana*, primarily for women. Though not actually a tonic itself, even in small amounts it catalyzes the tonic action of other herbs and promotes tissue growth in the reproductive organs and in the entire body. It can be added to milk or to other tonic herbs, like *shatavari* or angelica, to facilitate their function or used as a spice to promote assimilation of food into deeper tissues. Its quality is *sattvic* and gives energy to love, devotion and compassion, to *Bhakti Yoga*.

SAFFLOWER, sometimes misleadingly called saffron, can be used as a substitute for saffron and is much less expensive. It should be used in normal dosages.

SAGE   *Salvia officinalis; Labiatae*

Part Used: herb
Energetics: pungent, bitter, astringent/heating (slightly)/pungent
           KV– P+ (in excess)

Tissues: plasma, blood, nerve
Systems: respiratory, digestive, nervous, circulatory
Actions: diaphoretic, expectorant, nervine, astringent, alterative, diuretic, carminative, antispasmodic
Indications: colds, flus, sore throat, laryngitis, swollen lymph glands, night sweats, spermatorrhea, hair loss, nervous dysfunction
Precautions: high *Vata* (excessive dryness), nursing mothers
Preparations: infusion (hot or cold), powder (250 to 500 mg)

SAGE has a strong action for reducing excess secretions in the body. It stops sweating, is a specific for night sweats. It dries up excess mucus from the nose and lungs, as well as excessive salivation. It suppresses mammary secretions and withholds seminal discharge. It also dries up sores and ulcers and stops bleeding. As such it is mainly for reducing high *Kapha*. Taken hot, it is diaphoretic and expectorant and is good for *Kapha* and *Vata*. Taken cold, it is astringent and diuretic and is better for *Pitta*.

For the brain and nervous system and promoting the growth of hair, it combines well with gotu kola or *bhringaraj*. Sage has a special power to clear emotional obstructions from the mind and promote calmness and clarity. It helps reduce excessive desires and passions. It is specific for calming the heart.

It makes a good gargle for sore throat and a good wash for bleeding sore.

SANDALWOOD   *Santalum album; Santalaceae*

(S) *Chandana*

Part Used: wood and volatile oil
Energetics: bitter, sweet, astringent/cooling/sweet
　　　　　　PV– K or *Ama*+ (in excess)
Tissues: plasma, blood, muscle, marrow and nerve, reproductive
Systems: circulatory, nervous, digestive
Actions: alterative, hemostatic, antiseptic, antibacterial, carminative, sedative, refrigerant
Indications: eye diseases, cystitis, urethritis, vaginitis, acute dermatitis, herpes zoster, bronchitis, palpitations, gonorrhea, sunstroke
Precautions: high *Kapha*, severe lung congestion

Preparation: infusion (hot or cold), decoction, powder (250 mg to 1 g), medicated oil

SANDALWOOD cools and calms the entire body and mind, with its influence spreading throughout the circulatory, digestive, respiratory and nervous systems. It relieves fever, thirst, burning sensation and stops sweating. A few drops of sandalwood oil applied to the third eye will relieve heat and thirst, and is good for fever or overexposure to the sun.

Sandalwood helps the awakening of intelligence. Its *prabhava* is to help open the third eye, to increase devotion and promote meditation. It also aids in the transmutation of sexual energy.

Sandalwood, a good addition to other formulas, reduces fever; it is good for almost any inflammatory conditions and for cleansing the blood. Externally, the oil or paste can be used for most infectious sores or ulcers. In short, sandalwood is a very good anti-*Pitta* medicine.

A strong sandalwood oil can be made by steeping four ounces of sandalwood powder in one pint of cold water overnight, adding to one pint coconut oil and cooking over a low flame (not boiling), until all the water evaporates.

SARSAPARILLA   *Smilax spp.; Liliaceae*

(S) *Dwipautra*

(C) Tu fu ling

Part Used: rhizome
Energetics: bitter, sweet/cooling (slightly)/sweet
PV–; does not increase K
Tissues: plasma, blood, marrow and nerve, reproductive
Systems: circulatory, urinary, reproductive, nervous
Actions: alterative, diuretic, diaphoretic, antispasmodic, antisyphilitic, antirheumatic
Indications: venereal diseases, herpes, skin diseases, arthritis, rheumatism, gout, epilepsy, insanity, chronic nervous diseases, abdominal distention, intestinal gas, debility, impotence, turbid urine
Preparation: decoction, powder (250 mg to 1 g), paste, milk decoction

SARSAPARILLA purifies the urino-genital tract, dispelling all infection and inflammation. While purifying the blood, it also improves *Agni* and helps dispel accumulated *Vata* from the intestines. Its purifying action extends to the nervous system and it helps cleanse the mind of negative emotions; therefore, it is useful in many nervous disorders. Sarsaparilla's diaphoretic and blood-cleansing action is useful for rheumatic inflammation.

For herpes and venereal complaints, it can be combined with gentian. It stimulates the production of reproductive hormones and has tonic action on the sexual organs. As a blood-purifier it works well with burdock root. Externally, it can be used as a wash for genital sores or herpes, or as a hot fomentation for painful, arthritic joints.

SENNA   *Cassia acutifolia; Leguminosae*

(S) *Rajavriksha* (king of the trees)

(C) Fan xia ye

Part Used: leaves, pods (milder)
Energetics: bitter/cooling/pungent
　　　　　　PK– V+
Tissues: plasma, blood, fat
Systems: excretory, digestive, circulatory
Actions: purgative, anthelmintic, antipyretic, alterative
Indications: constipation, inflammatory skin conditions, hypertension, obesity
Precautions: hemorrhoids, inflammatory conditions of the g.i. tract, diarrhea, pregnancy
Preparation: infusion (hot or cold), powder (1 to 2 gms) as purgative

SENNA is a strong purgative that should be taken with care and in proper dosage. It has an irritant effect upon the intestinal membrane, and may cause griping, pain or nausea, along with liquid stools or diarrhea. It can be corrected by adding 1/4 amount of stomachic herbs, like ginger or fennel seeds, with its dosage.

Senna is mainly for severe constipation, the constipation following a fever, or for clearing *Pitta* from the small intestines (as in *virechana,* purgative therapy). However, it cannot be used where there is inflammation in the g.i. tract itself; not because it is heating, but because it is irritating. Except in conditions where rhubarb is not available or does not work, rhubarb is generally preferable to it and has fewer side effects.

Repeated use of strong purgatives, even of an herbal nature, may aggravate constipation and weaken the tone of the colon. Chronic constipation may be dealt with better by a moistening therapy and by laxative oils.

SESAME SEEDS   *Sesamum indicum; Pedaliaceae*

(S) *Tila*

(C) Hei chih ma

Part Used: seeds
Energetics: sweet/heating/sweet
          V– PK or *Ama*+ (in excess)
Tissues: works on all tissue-elements, particularly bone
Systems: respiratory, digestive, excretory, female reproductive
Actions: nutritive tonic, rejuvenative, demulcent, emollient, laxative
Indications: chronic cough, weak lungs, chronic constipation, hemorrhoids, dysentery, amenorrhea, dysmenorrhea, receding gums, tooth decay, hair loss, weak bones, osteoporosis, emaciation, convalescence
Precautions: obesity, high *Pitta*
Preparation: decoction, powder (500 mg to 2 gms), paste, medicated oil

SESAME SEEDS are a rejuvenative tonic for *Vata* constitution and for the bones and teeth. The black seeds are best, as they contain higher amounts of solar energy. A confection of the seeds can be made with one part sesame seeds, one-half part *shatavari* (if available), with ginger and raw sugar added to taste. One ounce of this mixture may be taken daily.

Sesame oil can be used in the same way as the seeds. It is similar in properties to olive oil. With equal parts of lime water, it can be applied externally for burns, boils and ulcers. Prepared with small amounts of camphor, cardamom and cinnamon, it can be applied to the head for migraines or vertigo. The powdered seeds can also be used externally as a paste.

Sesame seeds are *sattvic* and produce *sattvic* tissues in the body, and so are a good food for yogis, one ounce per day.

SKULLCAP *Scutellaria spp.; Labiatae*

Part Used: herb
Energetics: bitter/cooling/pungent
      PK– V+ (in excess)
Tissues: plasma, muscle, marrow and nerve
Systems: nervous, circulatory
Actions: nervine, antispasmodic, sedative, alterative
Indications: insomnia, convulsions, tremors, muscular spasms, neuralgia, epilepsy, neurosis, nervous headaches, hypertension, urinary and seminal incontinence, headaches, arthritis
Precautions: high *Vata*, deficient *Vata*, severe nerve deficiency
Preparation: infusion (hot or cold), powder (250 mg to 1 g)

SKULLCAP is a good calming herb that has special properties for lowering high *Pitta*, and for helping reduce the fiery emotions of anger, jealousy and hatred. It calms the heart and dispels excessive desire. It has a *sattvic* quality and promotes awareness, clarity and detachment. It allays excitability and restores control over deranged sensory and motor functions.

For improving awareness and promoting perception, it can be combined with gotu kola (1 teaspoon each per cup of hot water). As a nerve tonic it can be combined with *ashwagandha* in proportions of 1 to 4. Skullcap can be combined with bitter herbs like gentian for reducing *Pitta*.

SLIPPERY ELM *Ulmus fulva; Urticaceae*

Part Used: inner bark
Energetics: sweet/cooling/sweet
      VP– K and *Ama*+

Tissues: mainly plasma
Systems: respiratory, digestive
Actions: nutritive tonic, demulcent, expectorant, emollient, mild astringent
Indications: debility, convalescence, ulcers, hyperacidity, skin eruptions, burns, lung hemorrhage, weakness of lungs
Precautions: severe lung congestion, edema, high *Kapha*, high *Ama*
Preparation: decoction, powder (500 mg to 2 gms), powder, gruel, paste, milk decoction

SLIPPERY ELM is a highly nutritive, tonic herbal food for conditions of tissue deficiency. It helps rebuild the plasma element of the body, and helps restore the mucous membranes, particularly of the lungs and stomach. As such, it is good for recovery from chronic lung ailments, for desiccated lung tissue, dryness in the lungs, and for soothing and healing ulcerated membranes and surfaces.

Slippery elm is heavy, it may be hard to digest, and may promote congestion. As such, it is often wise to combine it with small amounts of spices such as cinnamon, cloves or ginger, or to sweeten it with honey. As a tonic, it can be decocted in milk, or with comfrey root and small amounts of licorice. For ulceration and hyperacidity, it can be used with small amounts of bitter stomachics, like gentian. Externally, the paste can be used to soothe burns, relieve inflammation and heal damaged tissue.

SOLOMON'S SEAL   *Polygonatum spp.; Liliaceae*

(S) *Meda, Mahmeda*

(C) Yu zhu

Part Used: rhizome
Energetics: sweet/cooling/sweet
          VPK= K or *Ama*+ (in excess)
Tissues: works on all tissue-elements, particularly blood, bone and reproductive
Systems: reproductive, respiratory, digestive
Actions: nutritive tonic, rejuvenative, aphrodisiac, demulcent, expectorant, hemostatic

Indications: debility, infertility, impotence, chronic bleeding disorders, diabetes, consumption, dry cough, dehydration, malnutrition, burning sensation, broken bones, inflamed mucous membranes
Precautions: severe congestion, high *Ama*
Preparation: decoction, milk decoction, powder (250 mg to 1 g), paste

Several different varieties of the Polygonatum species are used medicinally throughout the world, mainly for their demulcent and nutritive properties. There are European and American varieties as well as Indian and Chinese. All possess fairly similar powers. They are part of the many tonic and rejuvenative herbs of the lily family, including the onions and the lily itself. There is a special group of eight plant roots, *ashtavarga*, most in the lily family, famous in Ayurvedic medicine for promoting fertility, enhancing spermatogenesis, increasing lactation, and healing chronic wasting diseases like tuberculosis and weakness of the blood.

SOLOMON'S SEAL possesses demulcent and nutritive properties like slippery elm or comfrey root and can be used similarly. As a rejuvenative and aphrodisiac, it is superior. Taken internally, it helps heal broken bones. It is tonic to *Pitta* and *Vata* and to *shukra dhatu* (semen and reproductive tissue).

As a nutritive tonic, three grams of the powder may be taken twice a day mixed with warm milk and a teaspoon of *ghee* (clarified butter).

TURMERIC   *Curcuma longa; Zingiberaceae*

(S) *Haridra*

(C) Jiang huang

Part Used: rhizome
Energetics: bitter, astringent, pungent/heating/pungent
　　　　　K– PV+ (in excess)
Tissues: works on all tissue-elements in the body
Systems: digestive, circulatory, respiratory
Actions: stimulant, carminative, alterative, vulnerary, antibacterial
Indications: indigestion, poor circulation, cough, amenorrhea, pharyngitis, skin disorders, diabetes, arthritis, anemia, wounds, bruises

Precautions: acute jaundice and hepatitis, high *Pitta*, pregnancy
Preparation: infusion, decoction, milk decoction, powder (250 mg to 1 g)

TURMERIC is an excellent natural antibiotic, while at the same time it strengthens digestion and helps improve intestinal flora. As such it is a good antibacterial for those chronically weak or ill. It not only purifies the blood, but also warms it and stimulates formation of new blood tissue.

Turmeric gives the energy of the Divine Mother and grants prosperity. It is effective for cleansing the *chakras* (*nadi-shodhana*), purifying the channels of the subtle body. It helps stretch the ligaments and is, therefore, good for the practice of *hatha yoga*.

Turmeric promotes proper metabolism in the body, correcting both excesses and deficiencies. It aids in the digestion of protein.

Externally, it can be used with honey for sprains, strains, bruise or itch. It is tonic to the skin, for which purposes it can be taken internally as a milk decoction.

VALERIAN   *Valeriana spp.; Valerianaceae*

(S) *Tagara*

Part Used: rhizome
Energetics: bitter, pungent, sweet, astringent/heating/pungent
        VK– P+ (in excess)
Tissues: plasma, muscle, marrow and nerve
Systems: nervous, digestive, respiratory
Actions: nervine, antispasmodic, sedative, carminative
Indications: insomnia, hysteria, delirium, neuralgia, convulsions, epilepsy, vertigo, nervous cough, dysmenorrhea, palpitations, migraine, chronic skin diseases, flatulence, colic
Precautions: large dosages produce paralysis (overly constricts *Vata*)
Preparation: decoction (low simmer), powder (250 mg to 1 g)

VALERIAN is one of the best herbs for *Vatagenic* nervous disorders. It cleanses *Ama* from the colon, the blood, the joints and nerves. It clears the nerve channels of accumulated *Vata*. At the same time, owing to the large amounts of the earth element contained within it, it is grounding, and helps dispel vertigo, fainting and hysteria. Valerian calms muscle spasms and alleviates menstrual cramps. It is very effective for stopping fermentation in the gastrointestinal tract and has a special calming action on the female reproductive system. However, its quality is *tamasic* and excessive use can dull the mind.

It combines well with calamus, which balances out its heavy property. For sleep take one to two teaspoons of the powder in warm water.

WILD CHERRY BARK   *Prunus spp.; Rosaceae*

(S) *Padmaka*

Part Used: inner bark
Energetics: bitter, astringent/cooling/sweet
        PK– V+ (in excess)
Tissues: plasma, blood, muscle, marrow and nerve
Systems: respiratory, nervous, circulatory, digestive
Actions: expectorant, antispasmodic, alterative, astringent
Indications: cough, whooping cough, bronchial spasms, palpitations, skin problems, eye inflammation
Precautions: few, high *Vata*
Preparation: decoction, powder (250 to 500 mg), cough syrup

Various forms of wild cherry, apricot seeds and bitter almonds are effective expectorants and anticough agents, largely owing to the presence of hydrocyanic acid, which in large amounts is toxic. They cleanse and decongest the lungs and lymphatics. Those which are cooling, like wild cherry bark, extend this cleansing action to the blood. Apricot seeds and bitter almonds, however, owing to their oily properties as seeds, are heating in energy, as well as demulcent, emollient and laxative. They relieve a cough due to colds, but are only moderately effective on chronic coughs. It is this cleansing and expectorant action which causes apricot seeds to be used in anti-cancer therapy.

YARROW   *Achillea millefolium; Compositae*

(S) *Gandana*

(C) I chi kao

Part Used: leaves and flower-head
Energetics: bitter, astringent, pungent/cooling/pungent
              PK– V+ (in excess)
Tissues: plasma, blood, muscle
Systems: circulatory, respiratory, digestive
Actions: diaphoretic, astringent, hemostatic, vulnerary, antispasmodic
Indications: colds, fever, gastritis, enteritis, measles, menorrhagia, nosebleed, stomach ulcers, abcesses, hemoptysis
Precautions: high *Vata*
Preparation: infusion (hot or cold), powder (250 to 500 mg), paste

YARROW is a good cooling diaphoretic and febrifuge, which possesses astringent and antispasmodic properties. It is good for colds, flus and infectious diseases, particularly those in which fever and inflammation are high. It stops bleeding, both internally and externally. Yarrow reduces excessive menstrual bleeding and helps stop menstrual cramps. As such it is a good general herb for *Pitta* conditions, though its action is mild and mainly treats superficial conditions. Yarrow reduces excess *Pitta*, bile and inflammation in the gastrointestinal tract and thereby helps strengthen the mucous membranes. It has some calmative, nervine action and promotes clarity and perception.

Yarrow combines well with peppermint as a diaphoretic; with sage as an astringent and nervine; with chamomile (a relative of yarrow), as a stomachic.

Externally, the juice or decoction can be used as a wash for wounds and sores—mainly for stopping bleeding and reducing inflammation.

YELLOW DOCK   *Rumex crispus; Polygonaceae*

(S) *Amla vetasa*

Part Used: root
Energetics: bitter, astringent/cooling/pungent
        PK– V+
Tissues: plasma, blood
Systems: circulatory, urinary, lymphatic
Actions: alterative, astringent, laxative, antipyretic
Indications: toxic conditions of the blood, skin eruptions, swollen glands, glandular tumors, venereal diseases, hemorrhoids, stomach acidity
Precautions: emaciation, high *Vata*
Preparation: decoction, powder (250 to 500 mg)

YELLOW DOCK is a good general cleanser of blood and lymph, *rasa* and *rakta dhatus*; it is good for most toxic conditions of the circulatory system. A major herb for reducing high *Pitta*, it relieves toxic heat and clears infections, thereby reducing pain and inflammation. It contains large amounts of iron and can help build the blood, but it is mainly for a *Pitta*-kind of anemia (where bile thins the blood). In a *Vata*-kind of anemia, with chill and dryness in the blood, it will only cause further weakness. Yellow dock also has value in clearing and promoting cerebral circulation.

It is related to rhubarb root (also called *amla vetasa* in Sanskrit), which shares its properties, but is a stronger purgative. Together, and with other herbs, they can be used effectively for therapeutic purgation (*virechana*)—for cutting off accumulated *Pitta* at the root.

B. SPECIAL ORIENTAL HERBS

AJWAN, Wild Celery Seeds   *Apium graveolens; Umbelliferae*

(S) *Ajamoda*

Part Used: seeds
Energetics: pungent/heating/pungent
      KV– P+
Tissues: plasma, marrow and nerve
Systems: digestive, respiratory, nervous
Actions: stimulant, diaphoretic, expectorant, carminative, antispasmodic, diuretic, lithotriptic
Indications: colds, flus, laryngitis, bronchitis, asthma, cough, colic, indigestion, edema, arthritis
Precautions: hyperacidity, high *Pitta*
Preparation: infusion, powder (250 to 500 mg)

AJWAN or wild celery seed is a strong digestive, respiratory and nerve stimulant. For those suffering from high *Vata*, poor appetite, intestinal gas and sinus congestion, it may be taken as a powder, one to three grams three times a day before meals. It also promotes kidney function and energizes the nerves. Its uses are similar to wild carrot seeds in western herbalism. *Ajwan* is a powerful decongestant for both the respiratory and digestive tracts. It clears out deep-seated *Ama* and revives obstructed and stagnant metabolic functioning. It relieves intestinal spasms and vitalizes *Prana, samana* (the *Vata* governing digestion) and *udana* (the *Vata* governing speech, effort and enthusiasm). As such it helps improve aspiration and catalyze the ascending energies of the psyche.

DIAGRAM 9   *Chakras*

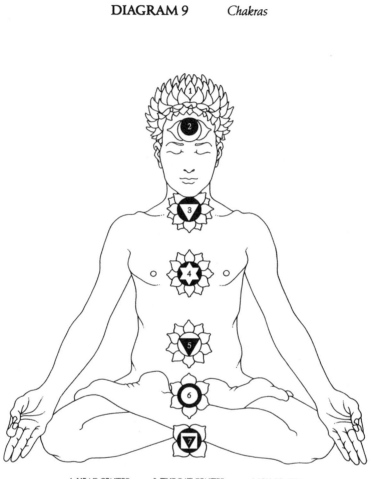

1. HEAD CENTER	3. THROAT CENTER	6. SEX CENTER
Calamus	*Apuan*	Coriander
Gotu Kola	Bayberry	*Gokshura*
Nutmeg	Cloves	Marshmallow
Valerian	Licorice	Uva Ursi
2. THIRD EYE	4. HEART CENTER	7. ROOT CENTER
Basil	Cardamom	*Ashwagandha*
Elecampane	Lotus Seeds	*Haritaki*
Sandalwood	Rose	Lotus Root
Skullcap	Saffron	*Shatavari*
	5. NAVEL CENTER	
	Black Pepper	
	Cayenne	
	Cumin	
	Golden Seal	

AMLA or *AMALAKI*, Emblic Myrobalan   *Emblica officinalis; Euphorbiaceae*

(S) *Amalaki* or *Dhatri*, the nurse, as it is like a nurse or mother in its healing properties

Part Used: fruit

Energetics: all tastes but salty, predominately sour/cooling/sweet
          PV– K and *Ama*+ (in excess)

Tissues: works on all tissue-elements and increases *Ojas*

Systems: circulatory, digestive, excretory

Actions: nutritive tonic, rejuvenative, aphrodisiac, laxative, refrigerant, stomachic, astringent, hemostatic

Indications: bleeding disorders, hemorrhoids, anemia, diabetes, gout, vertigo, gastritis, colitis, hepatitis, osteoporosis, constipation, biliousness, weakness of liver or spleen, premature greying or hair loss, convalescence from fever, general debility and tissue-deficiency, mental disorder, palpitation

Precautions: acute diarrhea, dysentery

Preparation: decoction, powder (250 mg to 1 g), confection

DIAGRAM 10   *Amalaki*

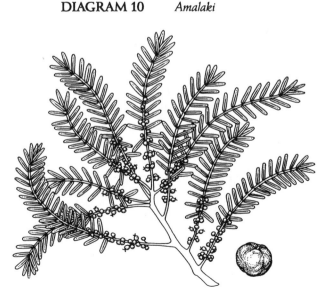

AMALAKI is one of the strongest rejuvenatives in Ayurvedic medicine. It is particularly effective as a *rasayana* for *Pitta*; for the blood, bones, the liver and the heart. It rebuilds and maintains new tissues and increases red blood cell count. *Amalaki* cleanses the mouth, strengthens the teeth, nourishes the bones, and causes hair and nails to grow. It improves the eyesight, stops bleeding of gums, and relieves inflammation of the stomach and colon. It is the highest natural source of vitamin C, with 3000 mg per fruit. It improves appetite, cleanses the intestines and regulates blood-sugar.

It is the basis for *CHYAVAN PRASH*, an herbal confection or jelly, that is the main general all-around tonic and restorative in Ayurvedic medicine. It is *sattvic* in quality and gives good fortune, love and longevity—it is itself a long-living tree. Five grams of the powder, mixed in one cup of warm water, can be taken twice a day as a general tonic. It is used as a paste to the head for mental disorders.

ANGELICA   *Angelica spp.; Umbelliferae*

(S) *Choraka*

(C) Dang gui (commonly called "Tang Kuei" or "Dong Quai")

Part Used: Root
Energetics: pungent, sweet/heating/sweet
            VPK= P+ (in excess)
Tissues: plasma, blood, muscle, marrow and nerve, reproductive
Systems: circulatory, female reproductive, respiratory, digestive
Actions: tonic, emmenagogue, rejuvenative, diaphoretic, antispasmodic, analgesic
Indications: amenorrhea, dysmenorrhea, menstrual cramps, P.M.S., anemia, headaches, colds, flus, arthritis, rheumatic pain
Precautions: hypertension, high *Pitta* conditions generally, use with care during pregnancy
Preparation: decoction, milk decoction, powder (250 mg to 1g), paste

A number of angelicas are used medicinally throughout the world. All possess diaphoretic and antirheumatic properties. Some also have tonic action on the blood and female reproductive system. The Chinese variety, tang kwei, and the Indian Angelica glauca, have strong tonic properties, which the European angelica possesses only to a lesser degree.

ANGELICA is one of the best tonics for women, nurturing the uterine organs and promoting their regular function. It is perhaps the best herb for regulating the menstrual cycle. As a tonic it works best with *shatavari*. For promoting menstruation it works well with safflower or saffron.

Both its tonic and antiarthritic actions are enhanced by small amounts of myrrh. Angelica promotes circulation and can be used externally for wounds, ulcers, itching and to nourish and beautify the skin. It is a good rejuvenative for women and works particularly well on *Vata* individuals.

One ounce of the root can be simmered in three cups of water for thirty minutes along with a little fresh ginger. It can be taken one day a week as a uterine tonic.

ASAFOETIDA   *Ferula asafoetida; Umbelliferae*

(S) *Hingu*

(C) A wei

Part Used: resin (exudate from the root)
Energetics: pungent/heating/pungent
        VK– P+
Tissues: plasma, blood, muscle, bone, marrow and nerves
Systems: digestive, nervous, respiratory, excretory, circulatory
Actions: stimulant, carminative, antispasmodic, analgesic, anthelmintic, aphrodisiac, antiseptic
Indications: indigestion, flatulence, abdominal distention, intestinal colic pain, constipation, arthritis, rheumatism, whooping cough, convulsions, epilepsy, hysteria, palpitation, asthma, paralysis, worms
Precautions: high fever, hyperacidity, rash, urticaria, pregnancy
Preparation: mainly powder (low dosage, 100 to 250 mg), paste

ASAFOETIDA is a powerful digestive agent, which removes food stagnation from the g.i. tract. It is effective in breaking up impacted fecal matter, accumulations from excessive eating of meat or junk food, and for destroying worms, particularly round worms and thread worms. Asafoetida cleanses the intestinal flora while strengthening *Agni*. It also dispels intestinal gas, relieves cramping and pain and subdues high *Vata*. It is similar in properties to garlic but stronger and more malodorous. You may have to put it in an air-tight jar or it will impart its sulphurous odor to the entire kitchen.

Externally, asafoetida can be applied as a paste for abdominal pain, arthritic pain, painful joints. As a spice, particularly for lentils and beans, it makes food lighter and decreases gas.

Like garlic, its quality is *tamasic*. It has a grounding but dulling effect upon the mind. It is used with such spices as ginger, cardamom and rock salt as a digestive agent. For dual action of stimulating *Agni* and moving *Vata* (*samana vayu*), there is probably nothing as effective. Like black pepper or cayenne, it should be found in every kitchen.

ASHWAGANDHA, Winter Cherry   *Withania somnifera;* *Solanaceae*

(S) *Ashwagandha*, that which has the smell of a horse, as it gives the vitality and sexual energy of a horse

Part Used: root
Energetics: bitter, astringent, sweet/heating/sweet
            VK– P and *Ama* + (in excess)
Tissues: muscle, fat, bone, marrow and nerve, reproductive
Systems: reproductive, nervous, respiratory
Actions: tonic, rejuvenative, aphrodisiac, nervine, sedative, astringent
Indications: general debility, sexual debility, nerve exhaustion, convalesence, problems of old age, emaciation of children, loss of memory, loss of muscular energy, spermatorrhea, overwork, tissue deficiency, insomnia, paralysis, multiple sclerosis, weak eyes, rheumatism, skin afflictions, cough, difficult breathing, anemia, fatigue, infertility, glandular swelling
Precautions: high *Ama*, severe congestion
Preparation: decoction, milk decoction, powder (250 mg to 1 g), paste, medicated *ghee*, medicated oil

ASHWAGANDHA holds a place in the Ayurvedic pharmacology similar to ginseng in Chinese medicine, yet it is far less expensive. It is the best rejuvenative herb, particularly for the muscles, marrow and semen and for *Vata* constitution. It is used in all conditions of weakness and tissue deficiency in children, the elderly, those debilitated by chronic diseases, those suffering from overwork, lack of sleep or nervous exhaustion.

For such regenerative purposes, it can be taken as a milk decoction to which may be added raw sugar, honey, *pippali* and *basmati* rice. As such, it inhibits aging and catalyzes the anabolic processes of the body. *Sattvic* in quality, it is one of the best herbs for the mind upon which it is nurturing and clarifying. It is calming and promotes deep, dreamless sleep.

Ashwagandha is a good food for weak pregnant women; it helps to stabilize the fetus. It also regenerates the hormonal system, promotes healing of tissues, and can be used externally on wounds, sores, etc. Five grams of the powder can be taken twice a day in warm milk or water, sweetened with raw sugar.

DIAGRAM 11   *Ashwagandha*

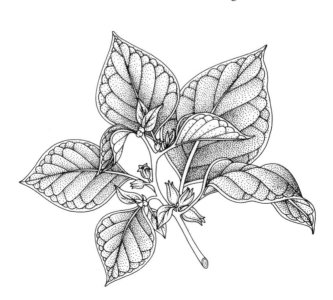

BALA, Indian Country Mallow   *Sida cordifolia; Malvaceae*

(S) *Bala,* what gives strength, owing to its strong tonic properties

Part Used: mainly root
Energetics: sweet/cooling/sweet
      VPK= K and *Ama*+ (in excess)
Tissues: works on all tissue-elements, especially marrow or nerve tissue
Systems: circulatory, nervous, urinary, reproductive
Actions: tonic, rejuvenative, aphrodisiac, demulcent, diuretic, stimulant, nervine, analgesic, vulnerary
Indications: heart disease, facial paralysis, sciatica, insanity, neuralgia, rheumatism, asthma, emaciation, exhaustion, sexual debility, cystitis, dysentery, leucorrhea, chronic fevers, convalescence
Precautions: few, congestive disorders of high *Ama* or *Kapha*
Preparation: decoction, milk decoction, powder (250 mg to 1 g), paste, medicated oil

Ayurvedic medicine uses several varieties of the Mallow family (like marshmallow) as tonics, demulcents and rejuvenatives. These include *bala, mahabala* (Sida rhombifolia), and *atibala* (Abutilon indicum), as well as Cotton Root, the root of the cotton plant. Though they all possess similar properties, *bala* is a more effective heart tonic, and *atibala* is a stronger diuretic, while cotton root is heating and is a stronger emmenagogue.

BALA is a tonic and *rasayana* for all kinds of *Vata* disorders. It feeds the nerves and is soothing for arthritic pain. It is also rejuvenative, nutritive and a stimulant to the heart. For deep seated, intermittent fevers, it can be given with ginger or black pepper. It relieves inflammation of nerve tissue.

Externally, as a medicated oil, it is good for nerve pain and numbness, and its softening action dispels muscle cramps. As a milk decoction with sugar, it is a good nutritive and aphrodisiac. It promotes healing of tissue in chronic infectious diseases.

BHRINGARAJ   *Eclipta alba, etc.; Compositae*

(S) *Bhringaraja, Kesharaja*, "ruler of the hair," as it promotes growth of
head hair

(C) Han lian cao

Part Used: herb
Energetics: bitter, pungent/heating/pungent
                 VK– increases *Pitta* only in excess
Tissues: plasma, blood, bone, marrow, reproductive
Systems: circulatory, nervous, digestive
Actions: tonic, rejuvenative, alterative, hemostatic, antipyretic, ner-
vine, laxative, vulnerary
Indications: premature greying of hair, balding, alopecia, loose or fall-
ing teeth, enlargement of liver and spleen, cirrhosis, chronic hepatitis,
bleeding, dysentery, anemia, skin diseases, insomnia, mental disorders
Precautions: severe chills
Preparation: infusion (hot or cold), decoction, powder (250 mg to
1 g), medicated oil, medicated *ghee*

BHRINGARAJ is a preventative to the aging process which maintains
and helps rejuvenate bones, teeth, hair, sight, hearing, and memory.
It is rejuvenative for the liver and an excellent medicine for
cirrhosis. It is also the best Ayurvedic herbal medicine for
the hair. *Bhringaraj* oil is famous for making the hair black and luxuriant; for removing greyness and reversing balding. It helps calm the
mind from excessive activity and promotes sound sleep.

In many respects it is similar to *brahmi*, or gotu kola, in its properties. It
combines the properties of a bitter tonic like dandelion (for which it is
a substitute) with a rejuvenative tonic.

Applied externally, it helps draw out poisons and reduces inflammation and swollen glands. It is a good tonic for the mind. *Bhringaraj* also
is good for the complexion. *Bhringaraj* grows wild in the southwestern
United States.

BIBHITAKI, Beleric Myrobalan

Terminalia belerica;
Combretaceae

(S) *Bibhitaki*

Part Used: fruit
Energetics: astringent/heating/sweet
        KP– V+ (in excess)
Tissues: plasma, muscle, bone
Systems: respiratory, digestive, excretory, nervous
Actions: astringent, tonic, rejuvenative, expectorant, laxative, anthelmintic, antiseptic, lithotriptic
Indications: cough, sore throat, laryngitis, bronchitis, catarrh, stones, chronic diarrhea, dysentery, parasites, eye diseases
Precautions: high *Vata*
Preparation: infusion, decoction, powder (250 mg to 1 g), paste

BIBHITAKI is another powerful rejuvenative herb of the various myrobalan trees which are widely used in India. It is tonic to *Kapha*, to the lungs; it improves voice, vision, and promotes the growth of hair. It is both strongly laxative and strongly astringent, cleansing the bowels and increasing their tone. *Bibhitaki* is effective for all manner of stones and *Kapha* accumulations in the digestive, urinary and respiratory tract; it liquifies and expels them, including removal of parasites. It astringes and tones the stomach and increases appetite. Though it is heating in energy, it does not aggravate *Pitta*.

As a powder mixed with honey, it can be taken for sore throat and impaired voice; it may also be used as a gargle. Used externally, it is an antiseptic. Usually, it is used as part of the compound *triphala* (see *haritaki*).

CHRYSANTHEMUM   *Chrysanthemum indicum; Compositae*

(S) *Sevanti*, service, as it gives the energy of devotion, surrender and service to the Divine

(C) Ju hua

Part Used: flowers

DIAGRAM 12   *Bibhitaki*

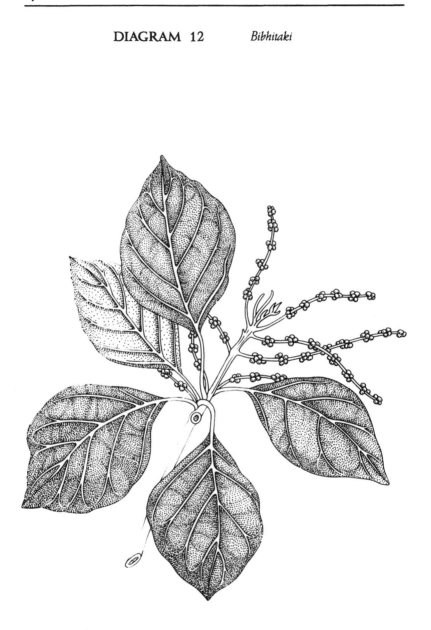

Energetics: bitter, sweet/cooling/pungent
       PK– V+ (in excess)
Tissues: plasma, blood, marrow
Systems: digestive, respiratory, nervous
Actions: diaphoretic, antipyretic, alterative, antispasmodic
Indications: headache, sore throat, eye infections, nose bleeds, boils, dysmenorrhea, liver diseases
Precautions: few, high *Vata*
Preparation: infusion (hot or cold), powder (250 mg to 1 g)

The common CHRYSANTHEMUM flower grown in gardens is a good cooling tea for summer heat or for *Pitta*-constitution individuals. Two teaspoons of the flowers may be steeped per cup of water. Chrysanthemum brightens the eyes and improves the vision, and is an important ingredient in many formulas for eye diseases. It cools and regulates the *Pitta* that governs vision. It calms *Pittogenic* emotions like anger and irritability. Soothing liver function, it helps promote menstruation, as it relieves menstrual cramps and headaches. It also works to promote lactation.

Chrysanthemum is an important flower in *Puja* (devotional worship). It aids in the surrender of the egoistic will (a function of deranged *Pitta*) to the Divine.

EPHEDRA   *Ephedra vulgaris; Gnetaceae*

(S) *Somalata,* from its similarities to soma as a strong stimulant to the nervous system

(C) Ma huang

Part Used: branches
Energetics: pungent, astringent/heating/pungent
       K– P+ V+ (in excess)
Tissues: plasma, muscle, marrow and nerve
Systems: respiratory, nervous, circulatory, urinary
Actions: stimulant, diaphoretic, expectorant, antispasmodic, diuretic, analgesic

Indications: colds, cough, dyspnea, wheezing, bronchitis, asthma, arthritis, dropsy, facial edema
Precautions: hypertension, cardiac pain, palpitations, insomnia, weak digestion
Preparation: infusion, powder (250 to 500 mg), use low dosages unless certain it has no side effects

EPHEDRA is probably the strongest stimulant and diaphoretic herb. It has an action like adrenaline. It can be used as a substitute for coffee, but is also has side effects (reduced somewhat by the addition of licorice to it). It may overstimulate the adrenals and burn out the nerves by its *rajasic* quality.

Ephedra is a powerful bronchodilator and is the source of ephedrine, one of the main medicines for asthmatic attacks. Yet it also may cause heart spasms. It is one of the most powerful *Kapha* reducing herbs, relieving cold, mucus, cough and edema, and promoting wakefulness and activity. It is used in many stimulant herbal blends and strongly stimulates the nerves. It relieves joint pain, promotes peripheral circulation and cleanses the lymphatics. It may be used with other milder diaphoretics like cinnamon and ginger.

AMERICAN EPHEDRA, also called Mormon tea, Brigham tea or joint fir, does not possess these same diaphoretic and anti-cough properties as the oriental variety. It is more commonly used as a diuretic, somewhat like juniper berries.

FO-TI   *Polygonum multiflorum; Polygonaceae*

(C) He shou wu

Part Used: root (processed)
Energetics: sweet, bitter, astringent/cooling/sweet
          PV– K and Ama + (in excess)
Tissues: works on all tissue-elements
Systems: reproductive, urinary, circulatory
Actions: tonic, rejuvenative, aphrodisiac, astringent, nervine
Indications: anemia, neurasthenia, impotence, lower back pain, premature greying or falling of the hair, enlarged lymph glands, excessive

menstruation, leucorrhea, arteriosclerosis, diabetes
Precautions: weak digestion, severe congestion or edema
Preparation: decoction, milk decoction, powder (250 mg to 1 g)

FO-TI is an important Chinese rejuvenative herb that is commonly
available in this country. It builds the blood and sperm and
strengthens the muscles, tendons, ligaments and bones. It strengthens
the kidneys, the liver and the nervous system and is a famous restorative for the hair. In terms of Ayurveda it is rejuvenative for *Pitta* and
Vata, and can be used in place of Ayurvedic tonics that are still largely
unavailable here.

Fo-ti is often combined with gotu kola, which brings together one of
the most important Chinese rejuvenatives with one of the most
important Indian. Both are used to counter the effects of aging; fo-ti is
better for rebuilding tissues; gotu kola is better for revitalizing the
mind.

One-half ounce of fo-ti can be simmered for thirty minutes in one
pint of water and taken daily. Or equal amounts of fo-ti and gotu kola
can be taken along with a small amount of fennel seeds to facilitate
their absorption.

GINSENG   *Panax ginseng; Araliaceae*

(C) Ren shen

Part Used: root
Energetics: pungent, bitter, sweet/heating/sweet
         VPK= PK+ (in excess)
Tissues: works on all tissue-elements of the body
Systems: digestive, respiratory, circulatory, nervous, reproductive
Actions: tonic, rejuvenative, stimulant, aphrodisiac, demulcent,
nervine
Indications: old age, senility, debility, emaciation, fatigue, impotence,
convalescence, to improve energy
Precautions: high blood pressure, fever, inflammatory conditions,
high *Pitta*, high *Ama* conditions generally, may overstimulate *Vata* in
excess, obesity
Preparation: decoction, milk decoction, powder (250 to 500 mg)

GINSENG is one of the best tonic and rejuvenative herbs, promoting growth and revitalization of the body and mind. It works particularly well for *Vata* disorders of tissue-deficiency found in old age. Those who are not weak may find it a stimulant, like coffee. It is excellent for promoting weight and tissue-growth in the body (including nerve tissue).

For rejuvenative purposes, it combines well with *ashwagandha*, an Indian herb of similar properties, when taken three grams twice a day. With ginger, it can be used to promote digestion and assimilation. It is a good general tonic cooked in milk.

American ginseng has similar properties but is said to be cooler in energy. It is a better demulcent and tonic to the lungs; better for *Pitta* individuals, but more likely to aggravate *Kapha*. American ginseng from the northern part of the country, the Catskills, however, is hotter and more like the Korean. The American variety is not inferior to the Chinese and we should make better use of it.

GOKSHURA, Caltrops   *Tribulis terrestris; Zygophyllaceae*

(S) *Gokshura, Shvadamstra*

(C) Chi li

Part Used: fruit
Energetics: sweet, bitter/cooling/sweet
          VPK=
Tissues: plasma, blood, marrow and nerve, reproductive
Systems: urinary, reproductive, nervous, respiratory
Actions: diuretic, lithotriptic, tonic, rejuvenative, aphrodisiac, nervine, analgesic
Indications: difficult or painful urination, edema, kidney or bladder stones, chronic cystitis, nephritis, hematuria, gout, rheumatism, lumbago, sciatica, impotence, infertility, seminal debility, venereal diseases, cough, dyspnea, hemorrhoids, diabetes
Precautions: dehydration
Preparation: decoction, milk decoction, powder (250 mg to 1 g), medicated oil

GOKSHURA is effective in most urinary tract disorders because it promotes the flow of urine, cools and soothes the membranes of the urinary tract, and aids in the discharge of stones. It stops bleeding, strengthens kidney function, while at the same time, nourishing the kidneys. As such, it is a rejuvenative tonic for the kidneys. It also strengthens the reproductive system by increasing semen; it is invigorating to postpartum women. *Gokshura* is rejuvenative to *Pitta*; at the same time, calming *Vata* with a sedative effect upon the nervous system. It is free of the side effects of most diuretics, and is somewhat similar in properties to marshmallow. It is a good harmonizing herb for most kidney formulas. It is *sattvic* in nature and promotes clarity.

Taken as a milk decoction it is a strong aphrodisiac. With equal amounts of dry ginger, it relieves nerve and back pain. With equal amounts of *ashwagandha* powder, three grams twice a day, it is a powerful revitalizer. The oil is good for alopecia and premature balding.

Gokshura is a common weed in the United States called Goat's Head or Puncture Vine, whose powerful medicinal qualities appear unknown here.

Another important tonic and rejuvenative for the kidneys is *punarnava* (Boerhaavia diffusa). It is usually used with *gokshura* in diuretic formulas.

GOTU KOLA   *Centella asiatica; Umbelliferae*

Part Used: herb
Energetics: bitter/cooling/sweet
          VPK=
Tissues: all tissue-elements but reproductive, mainly blood, marrow and nerve
Systems: nervous, circulatory digestive
Actions: nervine, rejuvenative, alterative, febrifuge, diuretic
Indications: nervous disorders, epilepsy, senility, premature aging, hair loss, chronic and obstinate skin conditions, venereal diseases

Precautions: may aggravate itching, in large doses may cause headaches or temporary loss of consciousness
Preparation: infusion (hot or cold), decoction, milk decoction, powder (250 to 500 mg), medicated *ghee*, medicated oil

GOTU KOLA is a close relative of *Brahmi* (*Hydrocotyle asiatica*) and is often used in the West as a substitute for it, for which it generally functions quite well, though with better diuretic and not quite as strong nervine properties. The herb increases intelligence, longevity, and memory. It fortifies the immune system, both cleansing and feeding it, and strengthens the adrenals. At the same time, it is a powerful blood purifier and is specific for chronic skin diseases, including leprosy and syphilis, as well as eczema and psoriasis. It is valuable in intermittent or periodic fevers, like malaria. *Gotu kola* is a tonic for *Pitta*. At the same time it inhibits *Vata*, calms the nerves, and helps reduce excessive *Kapha*. Note also section under *Brahmi*.

DIAGRAM 13
Gotu Kola

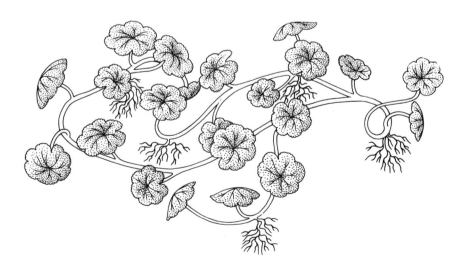

GUGGUL, Indian Bedellium   *Commiphora mukul; Burseaceae*

(S) *Guggulu*

Part Used: resin
Energetics: bitter, pungent, astringent, sweet/heating/pungent
         KV– P+ (in excess)
Tissues: works on all tissue-elements
Systems: nervous, circulatory, respiratory, digestive
Actions: rejuvenative, stimulant, alterative, nervine, antispasmodic,
analgesic, expectorant, astringent, antiseptic
Indications: arthritis, rheumatism, gout, lumbago, nervous disorders,
neurasthenia, debility, diabetes, obesity, bronchitis, whooping cough,
dyspepsia, hemorrhoids, pyorrhea, skin diseases, sores and ulcers, cystitis, endometritis, leucorrhea, tumors
Precautions: acute kidney infections, acute stage of rashes
Preparation: pill, powder (250 to 500 mg), paste

GUGGUL is the most important resin used in Ayurvedic medicine.
Similar to myrrh, it possesses strong purifying and rejuvenating
powers. A whole series of medicines, called *gugguls*, consist mainly of
this herb, with smaller amounts of other herbs used to direct its healing properties. It is a rejuvenative for *Vata*, and also for *Kapha*; it only
mildly aggravates *Pitta* after long term usage.

Guggul increases white blood cell count and disinfects secretions,
including mucus, sweat and urination. It increases appetite, clears the
lungs, and helps heal the skin and mucous membranes—though it is

DIAGRAM 14
Guggul

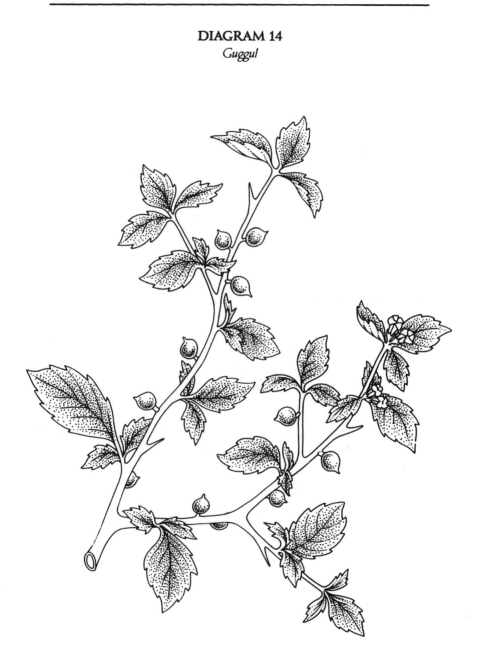

more for chronic than acute conditions. It can be applied externally as a plaster, as well as a gargle for ulcerated conditions of the mouth and throat. *Guggul* helps regulate menstruation. While not nutritive in itself, it does catalyze tissue regeneration, particularly nerve tissue. It also reduces fat, toxins, tumors and necrotic tissue. It is the best medicine for arthritic conditions.

HARITAKI, Chebulic Myrobalan   *Terminalia chebula;* Combretaceae

(S) *Haritaki,* because it carries away (*harate*) all diseases or because it is sacred to *Shiva* (*Hara*), also called *Abhaya* as it promotes fearlessness

(C) He zi (also the King of Medicines in Tibetan medicine)

Part Used: fruit
Energetics: all tastes but salty, predominantly
                astringent/heating/sweet
                VPK=
Tissues: works on all tissue elements
Systems: digestive, excretory, nervous, respiratory
Actions: rejuvenative, tonic, astringent, laxative, nervine, expectorant, anthelmintic
Indications: cough, asthma, hoarse voice, hiccough, vomiting, hemorrhoids, diarrhea, malabsorption, abdominal distention, parasitic infections, tumors, jaundice, spleen diseases, heart disease, skin diseases, itching, edema, nervous disorders
Precautions: pregnancy, dehydration, severe exhaustion or emaciation, in excess high *Pitta*
Preparation: decoction, powder (250 to 500 mg), paste

HARITAKI, though its taste is very astringent and unpleasant, is one of—if not the most—important Ayurvedic herb. It is a rejuvenative for *Vata,* regulating *Kapha* and only aggravating *Pitta* in excess. It feeds the brain and the nerves and imparts the energy of *Shiva* (pure awareness).

Haritaki is an effective astringent and gargle for ulcerated surfaces and membranes. It regulates the colon and, according to dosage, corrects either constipation or diarrhea. It improves digestion and absorption,

DIAGRAM 15
Haritaki

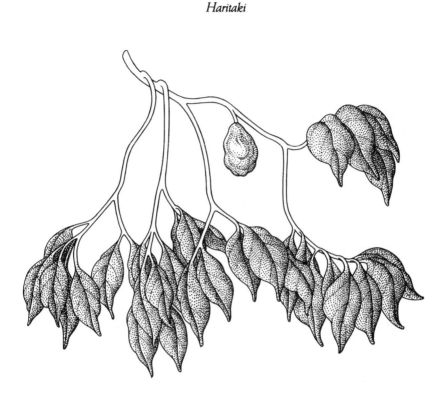

promotes voice and vision, and aids in longevity. *Haritaki* increases wisdom and intelligence.

It raises prolapse of the organs and checks excessive discharges, including cough, sweating, spermatorrhea, menorrhagia, and leucorrhea. It reduces accumulated and congested *Vata*.

Haritaki is the basis for *triphala*, the three fruits (*haritaki, amalaki* and *bibhitaki*), and is one of the main Ayurvedic compounds. *Triphala* is the best laxative and bowel tonic; a balanced *rasayana*, and an effective astringent for external use. *Haritaki* is rejuvenative for *Vata*; *amalaki* for *Pitta*; *bibhitaki* for *Kapha*. The conditions indicated under these three herbs can be treated by this compound.

JASMINE FLOWERS   *Jasminum grandiflorum; Oleaceae*

(S) *Jati*

Part Used: flowers
Energetics: bitter, astringent/cooling/pungent
        KP– V+ (in excess)
Tissues: plasma, blood, bone, marrow
Systems: nervous, circulatory, reproductive
Actions: alterative, refrigerant, antibacterial, hemostatic, emmenagogue, aphrodisiac, nervine
Indications: emotional disturbances, headaches, fever, sunstroke, conjunctivitis, dermatitis, burning urethra, bleeding disorders, bacterial or viral infections, cancer of lymph nodes, cancer of bones, Hodgkin's disease
Precautions: severe chills, high *Vata*
Preparation: infusion (hot or cold, do not boil), powder (250 to 500 mg), paste, medicated oil

JASMINE FLOWERS are strongly cooling and calming. Their blood-cooling effects include strong antibacterial, antiviral and antitumor action, through which they also stop bleeding. They strengthen the lymphatic system and are helpful in different kinds of cancer, including breast cancer. They are excellent for fevers and the oil helps relieve sunstroke.

Jasmine flowers are mildly aphrodisiac for the female and cleanse the uterus. *Sattvic* in quality they increase love and compassion. They carry psychic influences, make the mind receptive, aid, receive and radiate the vibrations of *mantras*. They combine well with sandalwood for most purposes. They are also useful in high fevers from infectious and contagious diseases.

LOTUS   *Nelumbo nucifera; Nymphaeceae*

(S) *Padma, Kamala, Pushkara,* etc. Sanskrit abounds with many names for the lotus, India's most sacred plant and symbol of spiritual unfoldment

(C) Lian zi (seed), Ou jie (root)

Part Used: mainly seeds and root
Energetics: sweet, astringent/cooling/sweet
          PV− K+ (in excess)
Tissues: plasma, blood, marrow and nerve, reproductive
Systems: digestive, circulatory, reproductive, nervous
Actions: nutritive tonic, rejuvenative, aphrodisiac, astringent, hemostatic, nervine
Indications: diarrhea, bleeding disorders, menorrhagia, leucorrhea, impotence, spermatorrhea, venereal diseases, heart weakness
Precautions: *Ama* conditions, indigestion, food stagnation, constipation
Preparation: decoction, powder (250 mg to 1 g), food

LOTUS SEEDS and LOTUS ROOT are tonic and rejuvenating foods. The seeds work more as a cardiac tonic and as a seminal tonic. The root has stronger astringent and hemostatic properties and works more on first *chakra* disorders (diarrhea, hemorrhoids, etc.) as its quality is heavier. As a food, lotus seeds can be taken as a powder, five grams three times a day, with *basmati* rice or other tonics like *shatavari* and *ashwagandha*, suitably spiced and sweetened.

The lotus is sacred to *Lakshmi*, the goddess of prosperity, and brings material and spiritual abundance. It calms the mind and subdues restless thoughts and dreams. Lotus seeds help open the heart center; lotus root, the root center. The seeds are good for devotion and aspiration. They also improve speech, help stop stuttering and improve concentration.

Makhanna (Chinese foxnuts, Euyrale ferox) has similar properties and is often used together with lotus seeds. American white pond lily (water lily root) has similar properties to lotus root; it is a good astringent and hemostatic with the power to heal tumors.

MANJISHTA, Indian Madder   *Rubia cordifolia; Rubiaceae*

(S) *Manjishta*

(C) Qian cao

Part Used: root

Energetics: bitter, sweet/cooling/pungent
            PK– V+
Tissues: plasma, blood, muscles
Systems: circulatory, female reproductive
Actions: alterative, hemostatic, emmenagogue, astringent, diuretic, lithotriptic, antitumor
Indications: amenorrhea, dysmenorrhea, menorrhagia, menopause, bleeding disorders, kidney or bladder stones, gall stones, jaundice, hepatitis, diarrhea, dysentery, broken bones, traumatic injuries, cancer, heart disease, skin problems, dropsy, rickets, paralysis, herpes
Precautions: severe chills, high *Vata*
Preparation: decoction, powder (250 mg to 1 g), paste, medicated *ghee*

MANJISHTA is probably the best alterative or blood-purifying herb in Ayurvedic medicine. It cools and detoxifies the blood, arrests hemorrhage, dissolves obstructions in blood flow, and removes stagnant blood. Good for all inflammatory conditions of the blood (or the female reproductive system), its obstruction-dissolving action extends to the liver and kidneys. It dissolves stones and helps destroy tumors, benign or malignant. It increases blood flow and promotes healing of tissue damaged by injury or infection. *Manjishta* even helps knit broken bones; it is, therefore, a good first aid medicine. An effective medicine for toxic blood conditions (such as genital herpes), it cleanses and regulates liver, spleen and kidney function.

Externally, it can be used as a paste with honey for skin discoloration or skin inflammations. Or it can be made into a paste with licorice to soothe burned or damaged tissue. It is one of the main anti-*Pitta* herbs.

European madder (Rubia tinctorum) has similar properties and is a good substitute.

MUSTA, Nutgrass   *Cyperus rotundus; Cyperaceae*

(S) *Musta*

(C) Xiang fu

Part Used: rhizome
Energetics: pungent, bitter, astringent/cooling/pungent
            PK– V+ (in excess)

Tissues: plasma, blood, muscle, marrow and nerve
Systems: digestive, circulatory, female reproductive
Actions: stimulant, carminative, astringent, alterative, emmenagogue, antispasmodic, anthelmintic
Indications: menstrual disorders, dysmenorrhea, menopause, diarrhea, malabsorption, indigestion, sluggish liver
Precautions: constipation, high *Vata*
Preparation: decoction (low simmer), powder (250 mg to 1 g)

MUSTA is the Indian variety of the common nutgrass found in most marshy areas and river bottoms. It is one of the most important herbs for treating female disorders because it relieves menstrual pain, dispels premenstrual congestion of blood and water. It is one of the most effective menstrual regulators.

Musta is one of the best digestive stimulants for *Pitta* constitution and an effective stimulant for the liver. It improves absorption in the small intestine and thereby stops diarrhea, while at the same time helping to destroy parasites. As such it may be helpful in such problems as Candida, gastrointestinal yeast infections. It is effective in chronic fevers and for promoting digestion in such conditions as gastritis.

As an emmenagogue, it can be used with *shatavari* or tang kuei in proportions of 1 to 4, one ounce of the herbs simmered in one pint of water for twenty minutes. With ginger and honey it is a good all-purpose medicine for improving digestion. It is particularly good for the emotional problems of P.M.S., i.e. depression or irritability.

NEEM   *Azadiracta indica; Meliaceae*

(S) *Nimba*

Part Used: bark, leaves (available at most Indian markets)
Energetics: bitter/cooling/pungent
       PK– V+
Tissues: plasma, blood, fat
Systems: digestive, circulatory, respiratory, urinary
Actions: bitter tonic, antipyretic, alterative, anthelmintic, antiseptic, antiemetic
Indications: skin diseases (urticaria, eczema, ringworm), parasites,

fever, malaria, cough, thirst, nausea, vomiting, diabetes, tumors, obesity, arthritis, rheumatism, jaundice
Precautions: diseases of cold and tissue deficiency generally
Preparation: infusion (hot or cold), decoction, powder (250 to 500 mg), paste, medicated *ghee*, medicated oil

NEEM is one of the most powerful blood-purifiers and detoxifiers in Ayurvedic usage. It cools the fever and clears the toxins involved in most inflammatory skin diseases or those found in ulcerated mucous membranes. It is a powerful febrifuge, effective in malaria and other intermittent and periodic fevers (in which case it is usually used with black pepper and gentian).

Neem can be taken whenever a purification or reduction program is indicated. It clears away all foreign and excess tissue, and possesses a supplementary astringent action that promotes healing. Yet it should be used with discretion where there is severe fatigue or emaciation. In a medicated oil, it is one of the best healing and disinfectant agents for skin diseases, and anti-inflammatory agent for joint and muscle pain.

PIPPALI, Indian Long Pepper   *Piper longum; Piperaceae*

(S) *Pippali*

(C) Chinese: Bi bo

Part Used: fruit
Energetics: pungent/heating/sweet
        VK– P+
Tissues: plasma, blood, fat, marrow and nerve, reproductive
Systems: digestive, respiratory, reproductive
Actions: stimulant, expectorant, carminative, aphrodisiac, anthelmintic, analgesic
Indications: colds, coughs, asthma, bronchitis, laryngitis, arthritis, rheumatism, gout, dyspepsia, abdominal distention, flatulence, abdominal tumors, lumbago, sciatica, epilepsy, paralysis, worms
Precautions: high *Pitta* (inflammatory conditions)
Preparation: infusion, milk decoction, medicated oil, powder (100 to 500 mg)

DIAGRAM 16
Pippali

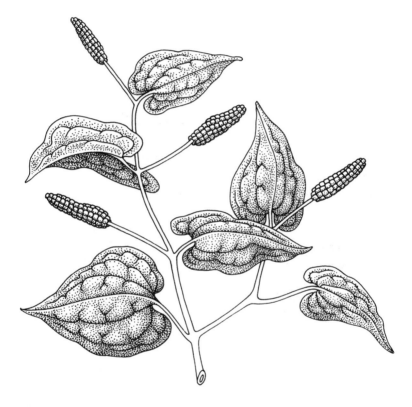

PIPPALI, like its close relative black pepper, is a powerful stimulant for both the digestive and respiratory systems. It is strongly heating and removes cold, congestion and *Ama,* and revives weakened organic functions. Unlike black pepper it is also a rejuvenative, mainly for the lungs and for *Kapha*. Prepared as a milk decoction, it can help cure chronic, degenerative lung diseases like asthma.

Pippali is also an aphrodisiac and strengthens reproductive functions, warming and energizing the reproductive organs. Three of the pods may be taken daily in the morning with a little honey to control excess secretions, mucus and *Kapha*. Alternatively, ten black peppercorns can be used.

Together with black pepper and dry ginger, *pippali* forms the compound known as *trikatu*, or the three spices. This is the main stimulant compound used in Ayurveda. *Trikatu* rejuvenates *Agni*, burns away *Ama* and allows for the assimilation of other medicines and foods.

REHMANNIA   *Rehmannia glutinosa; Scrophulariaceae*

(C) Di huang (cooked, Shu di huang)

Part Used: root
Energetics: sweet, bitter/cooling/sweet
            PV- K and *Ama* +
Tissues: plasma, blood, marrow and nerve, reproductive
Systems: reproductive, urinary, digestive, respiratory
Actions: nutritive tonic, rejuvenative, aphrodisiac, demulcent, laxative, emmenagogue
Indications: weak kidneys, low back pain, sexual debility (male or female), irregular menstruation, cirrhosis, anemia, hair loss, diabetes, senility
Precautions: weak digestion, severe congestion or edema
Preparation: mainly decoction, powder (250 mg to 1 g)

REHMANNIA is an important tonic and rejuvenative herb for the kidneys and liver, widely used in Chinese medicine. The raw form is used for clearing deep-seated fevers and is thought to be cooling in energy. The cooked form is used for most tonic purposes and is thought to be slightly warming.

In terms of Ayurveda, Rehmannia is *Kapha* in nature; it increases bodily tissues, fluids and secretions. Both kinds, raw and cooked, decrease *Pitta* and treat such *Pitta* disorders as anemia. Cooked rehmannia is a good substitute for *shatavari* as a tonic and rejuvenative for the uterus.

Cooked rehmannia is a major herb for the problems of aging and helps counter dryness and lack of vitality of high *Vata* conditions. Yet it is somewhat greasy and may need to be given along with digestion-increasing herbs like cinnamon or ginseng, so that it does not cause diarrhea. Five to ten grams can be simmered in a pint of water for thirty minutes and one cup can be taken before meals as a nutritive tonic.

SHATAVARI *Asparagus racemosus; Liliaceae*

(S) *Shatavari*, "who possesses a hundred husbands," as its tonic and rejuvenative action on the female reproductive organs is said to give the capacity to have a hundred husbands

(C) Tian men dong

Part Used: root
Energetics: sweet, bitter/cooling/sweet
            PV– K or *Ama+* (in excess)
Tissue: works on all tissue-elements
Systems: circulatory, reproductive, respiratory, digestive
Actions: tonic (general, reproductive and nervine), nutritive, rejuvenative, demulcent, antacid
Indications: debility of the female organs, sexual debility generally, infertility, impotence, menopause, diarrhea, dysentery, stomach ulcers, hyperacidity, dehydration, lung abscess, hematemesis, cough, convalescence, cancer, herpes, leucorrhea, chronic fevers
Precautions: high *Ama*, excessive mucus
Preparation: decoction, milk decoction, powder (250 mg to 1 g), paste, medicated *ghee*, medicated oil

SHATAVARI is the main Ayurvedic rejuvenative for the female–as is *ashwagandha* for the male (though both have some action on both sexes). It is a *rasayan* for *Pitta*, for the female reproductive system, and for the blood. As such, it can be prepared as a milk decoction, along with *ghee*, raw sugar, honey and *pippali*.

It is an effective demulcent for dry and inflamed membranes of the lungs, stomach, kidneys and sexual organs. As such, it is good for ulcers, and with its thirst-relieving and fluid-protecting powers it is good for chronic diarrhea and dysentery.

Externally, it is an effective emollient for stiff joints, stiff neck and muscle spasms. It soothes and calms *Vata*.

It increases milk, semen and nurtures the mucous membranes. It both nourishes and cleanses the blood and the female reproductive organs. It is a good food for menopause or for those who have had hysterectomies, as it supplies many female hormones. It nourishes the ovum and increases fertility, yet its quality is *sattvic* and aids in love and devotion. Three grams of the powder can be taken in one cup of warm milk sweetened with raw sugar.

Western asparagus root has some similar properties but is more diuretic.

DIAGRAM 17
Shatavari

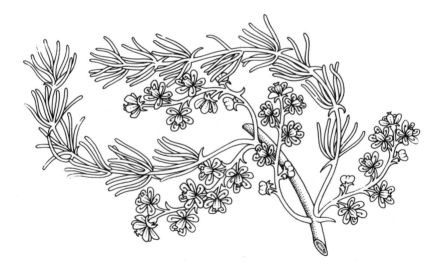

VAMSHA ROCHANA, Bamboo Manna   *Bambusa arundinaceae; Graminaceae*

(S) *Vamsha-rochana*

(C) Zhu ru

Part Used: the siliceous deposits or milky bark of the plant (sap may be used as substitute)
Energetics: sweet, astringent/cooling/sweet
            PV– K+
Tissues: plasma, blood, marrow and nerve
Systems: respiratory, circulatory, nervous
Actions: demulcent, expectorant, tonic, rejuvenative, antispasmodic, hemostatic
Indications: colds, cough, fever, asthma, bleeding disorders, emaciation, debility, dehydration, palpitation, vomiting, consumption
Precautions: may increase congestion if not balanced out by pungent herbs like ginger and *pippali.*
Preparation: decoction, milk decoction, powder (250 mg to 1 g)

The bamboo plant has extensive medicinal usages. The leaves and the milky inner bark of the plant, called *VAMSHA ROCHANA* or bamboo manna, have strong anti-*Pitta* properties that help conditions of lung weakness. It also stops bleeding and clears fever and cough.

Vamsha rochana is a rejuvenative for the lungs and an all-purpose moistening expectorant like comfrey root. With heating diaphoretics, it forms the basis for some of the major anti-cold and cough formulas in Ayurvedic medicine. At the same time, it is nourishing and helps increase vigor and strength for recovery from chronic diseases and for tissue-deficiency. It nurtures the heart and soothes the nervous system. It relieves thirst and anxiety and improves the blood.

WILD YAM   *Dioscorea spp.; Dioscoraceae*

(S) *Aluka*

(C) Shan yao

Part Used: root

Energetics: sweet, bitter/cooling/sweet
          VP– K+ (in excess)
Tissues: plasma, muscle, fat, marrow and nerve, reproductive
Systems: nervous, reproductive, digestive, urinary
Actions: nutritive tonic, aphrodisiac, rejuvenative, diuretic, antispasmodic, analgesic
Indications: impotency, senility, hormonal deficiency, infertility, colic, nervous excitability, hysteria, abdominal pain and cramps
Precautions: excess mucus in the body, congestion
Preparation: decoction, milk decoction, powder (250 mg to 1 g)

Many of the different varieties of WILD YAM possess strong rejuvenative powers (others do not, so be sure of the particular species). They increase semen, milk and other hormonal secretions, as well as promoting body weight. The American variety also contains many hormones and is an effective tonic for the female reproductive system. It is also used for its nervine and antispasmodic properties. Some of the oriental varieties, as well as the Mexican variety, are regarded as rejuvenatives for men. Wild yam also has a soothing and harmonizing effect upon the digestive organs.

VIDARI-KANDA (Ipomomea digitata), a relative of the sweet potato, is used similarly to the wild yam as an aphrodisiac, galactogogue and nutritive tonic. In fact, it is thought to have stronger properties in this regard. It has been called an "Indian ginseng."

PUERARIA, the kudzu plant (Pueraria tuberosa), is used as a substitute for arrowroot and is a common weed (an invasive vine) in the southern United States. It is sometimes used as a substitute for *vidari-kanda*, and also has some aphrodisiac properties. Both plants produce massive, starchy roots.

Five grams of the powder of wild yam, *vidari-kanda* or pueraria, can be cooked in a cup of milk with *ghee*, honey and raw sugar to taste, and taken daily as a restorative for seminal debility, deficient lactation or emaciation.

DIAGRAM 18
HERBS & THE ORGANS

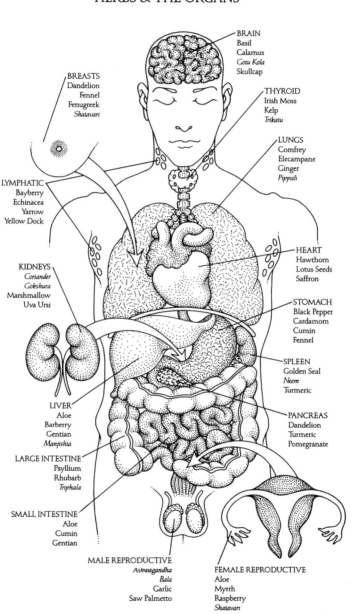

BREASTS
Dandelion
Fennel
Fenugreek
Shatavari

BRAIN
Basil
Calamus
Gotu Kola
Skullcap

THYROID
Irish Moss
Kelp
Trikatu

LUNGS
Comfrey
Elecampane
Ginger
Pippali

LYMPHATIC
Bayberry
Echinacea
Yarrow
Yellow Dock

HEART
Hawthorn
Lotus Seeds
Saffron

KIDNEYS
Coriander
Gokshura
Marshmallow
Uva Ursi

STOMACH
Black Pepper
Cardamom
Cumin
Fennel

SPLEEN
Golden Seal
Neem
Turmeric

LIVER
Aloe
Barberry
Gentian
Manjishta

PANCREAS
Dandelion
Turmeric
Pomegranate

LARGE INTESTINE
Psyllium
Rhubarb
Triphala

SMALL INTESTINE
Aloe
Cumin
Gentian

MALE REPRODUCTIVE
Ashwagandha
Bala
Garlic
Saw Palmetto

FEMALE REPRODUCTIVE
Aloe
Myrrh
Raspberry
Shatavari

APPENDICES

APPENDIX I

BEVERAGE TEAS FOR THE THREE DOSHAS

The use of herbal teas as beverages, as substitutes or alternatives for coffee or tea, has become very common. Yet without a proper understanding of constitution and condition, the use of such herbal teas may not be entirely health-promoting.

Below is a list of common herbs used as teas or general tonics. Other herbs that may be used as beverages should similarly be related according to constitution and condition so that their real effectiveness can manifest.

This is not to recommend all these herbs for general usage as beverages. Any herb you wish to take as a common beverage should be taken in low dosages and examined for possible long term effects.

KAPHA: Most herbal teas are good for *Kapha*, except those like licorice, which are sweet and mucus-forming.

Alfalfa, basil, blackberry, black pepper, burdock, cardamom, celery seeds, chamomile, cinnamon, cleavers, cloves, dandelion, eucalyptus, ginger, hawthorn, hyssop, juniper berries, lemon, Mormon tea, mustard seeds, nettle, orange peel, parsley, peppermint, sage, sassafras, skullcap, spearmint, sumach, thyme, wild carrot, wild ginger, yarrow, yellow dock

PITTA: Many herbal teas are good for *Pitta*, but those pungent or hot in energy should be avoided.

Alfalfa, blackberry, burdock, chamomile, chicory, chrysanthemum, comfrey, coriander, cumin, dandelion, fennel, gotu kola, hibiscus, jasmine, lemon, lemon balm, lemon grass, licorice, lime, marshmallow, motherwort, nettle, peppermint, raspberry, rose flowers, red clover, red root, saffron, sandalwood, skullcap, spearmint, strawberry, yellow dock

VATA: Many herbal teas are good for *Vata*, but those bitter, astringent or cold in energy may not be beneficial. Combinations of pungent and sweet herbs are best for *Vata*.

Anise, angelica, basil, bay leaves, cardamom, celery seeds, cinnamon, cloves, comfrey root, elecampane, eucalyptus, fennel, fenugreek, fo-ti, fresh ginger, ginseng, gotu kola, hawthorn, Irish moss, licorice, nutmeg, orange peel, rehmannia, safflower, sassafras, saw palmetto, sarsaparilla, Solomon's seal, thyme, wild ginger, yerba santa

SWEETENERS: *Kapha* constitution should avoid sweeteners in teas, except honey. All sweeteners are good for *Pitta*, except honey. All sweeteners are good for *Vata* and help balance out the *Vata*-increasing properties of some herbs. Refined sugar, however, should be avoided, as it overstimulates the pancreas.

Some teas good in moderation for all constitutions include chamomile, fennel, gotu kola, peppermint, rose flowers, sage, spearmint.

APPENDIX II   HERB CHART

Herbs are listed according to their common names. Taste is according to the six Ayurvedic tastes; sweet, sour, salty, pungent, bitter, astringent. Energy is heating or cooling. P-D effect is *vipaka* or post-digestive effect (sweet, sour or pungent). Action on *dosha*: V is *Vata*, P is *Pitta*, K is *Kapha*, + is increases, – is decreases, 0 is neutral or mixed in effect. VPK= is balancing to all three *doshas*. Therepeutic properties are according to western herbalism. Herbs starred are those also contained in the main text.

HERB	TASTE	ENERGY	PD-EFFECT	DOSHA	ACTIONS
AGRIMONY *Agrimonia eupatoria* *Rosaceae*	astringent, bitter	cooling	pungent	PK– V+	astringent, diuretic, vulnerary
***ALFALFA** *Medicago sativa* *Leguminosae*	astringent, sweet	cooling	pungent	PK– V+	alterative, diuretic, antipyretic
ALLSPICE *Pimento officinalis* *Myrataceae*	pungent	heating	pungent	VK– P+	stimulant, carminative
ALMOND *Amygdalus communis* *Rosaceae*	sweet	heating	sweet	V– KP+	demulcent, expectorant, tonic
***ALOE** *Aloe spp.* *Liliaceae*	bitter, astringent, pungent, sweet	cooling	sweet	VPK= (P–)	alterative, bitter tonic, rejuvenative, purgative
ANGELICA *Angelica archangelica* *Umbelliferae*	pungent, sweet	heating	sweet	VK– P+	diaphoretic, carminative, emmenagogue
ANISE *Pimpinella anisum* *Umbelliferae*	pungent	heating	pungent	VK– P+	carminative, stimulant, galactagogue
APRICOT SEED *Prunus armeniaca* *Rosaceae*	bitter, sweet	heating	pungent	KV– P+	antispasmodic, expectorant, laxative

Herb		heating/cooling		energetics	actions
ARNICA *Arnica montana* Compositae	pungent	heating	pungent	KV– P+	stimulant, vulnerary, tonic
ASPARAGUS *Asparagus officinalis* Liliaceae	sweet	cooling	sweet	PK– Vo	diuretic, laxative, tonic
BALMONY *Chelone glabra* Scrophulariaceae	bitter	cooling	pungent	PK– V+	bitter tonic, anthelmintic, laxative
***BARBERRY** *Berberis spp.* Berberidaceae	bitter, astringent	heating	pungent	PK–V+	bitter tonic, alterative, antipyretic
BARLEY *Hordeum distichon* Graminaceae	sweet	cooling	sweet	PK– V+	diuretic, demulcent, tonic
***BASIL** *Ocinum spp.* Labiatae	pungent	heating	pungent	VK–P+	diaphoretic, febrifuge, nervine
***BAYBERRY** *Myrica spp.* Myricaceae	pungent, astringent	heating	pungent	KV– P+	diaphoretic, expectorant, astringent, emetic
BAY LEAVES *Laurus nobilis* Lauraceae	pungent	heating	pungent	VK– P+	carminative, stimulant, expectorant

HERB	TASTE	ENERGY	PD-EFFECT	DOSHA	ACTIONS
BETONY, WOOD *Stachys betonica* *Labiatae*	pungent, bitter	cooling	pungent	PK– V+	nervine, carminative, diuretic
BIRCH *Betula alba* *Betulaceae*	bitter, pungent	cooling	pungent	PK– V+	diaphoretic, diuretic, astringent
BISTORT *Polygonum bistorta* *Polygonaceae*	astringent	cooling	pungent	PK– V+	astringent, diuretic, alterative
BITTER ROOT *Apocynum androsaemifolium* *Apocynaceae*	bitter, astringent	cooling	pungent	PK– V+	cathartic, emetic, diuretic
BLACKBERRY *Rubus fructicosus, etc.* *Rosaceae*	astringent	cooling	sweet	PK– V+	astringent, alterative, hemostatic
BLACK COHOSH *Cimicufuga* *Ranunculaceae*	bitter, pungent	cooling	pungent	PK– V+	alterative, emmenagogue, antiseptic
*BLACK PEPPER *Piper nigrum* *Piperaceae*	pungent	heating	pungent	KV– P+	stimulant, expectorant, carminative
BLESSED THISTLE *Carbenia benedicta* *Compositae*	bitter	cooling	pungent	PK– V+	emmenagogue, bitter tonic, galactagogue

Herb	Taste	Temperature		Dosha	Actions
BLUE COHOSH *Caulophyllum thalictroides* *Berberidaceae*	bitter, sweet	heating	pungent	KV – P+	emmenagogue, parturient, antispasmodic
BLUE FLAG *Iris versicolor* *Iridaceae*	bitter	cooling	pungent	PK – V+	alterative, antipyretic, laxative
BONESET *Eupatorium perfoliatum* *Compositae*	bitter, pungent	cooling	pungent	PK – V+	diaphoretic, antipyretic, laxative
BORAGE *Borago officinalis* *Boraginaceae*	astringent, sweet	cooling	pungent	PK – V+	diaphoretic, diuretic, demulcent
BUCHU *Barosma betulina* *Rutaceae*	pungent, bitter	cooling	pungent	PK – V+	diuretic, diaphoretic, stimulant
BUCKBEAN *Menyanthes trifoliata* *Gentianaceae*	bitter	cooling	pungent	PK – V+	alterative, antipyretic, laxative
*BURDOCK *Arctium lappa* *Compositae*	bitter, pungent	cooling	pungent	PK – V+	alterative, diaphoretic, diuretic, astringent
BUTTERNUT *Juglans cinerea* *Juglandacae*	bitter, astringent	cooling	pungent	PK – V+	purgative, anthelmintic, astringent

HERB	TASTE	ENERGY	PD-EFFECT	DOSHA	ACTIONS
*CALAMUS (Sweet Flag) *Acorus calamus* *Araceae*	pungent, bitter	heating	pungent	VK – P+	stimulant, decongestant, nervine, rejuvenative
CALENDULA *Calendula officinalis* *Compositae*	bitter, pungent	cooling	pungent	PK – V+	vulnerary, antispasmodic alterative
CALUMBA *Jateorhiza calumba* *menispermaceae*	bitter	cooling	pungent	PK – V+	bitter tonic, antipyretic, antiemetic
*CAMPHOR *Cinnamomum camphora* *Lauraceae*	pungent, bitter	heating	pungent	KV – P+	diaphoretic, stimulant, decongestant, analgesic
CARAWAY *Carum carvi* *Umbelliferae*	pungent	heating	pungent	KV – P+	carminative, stimulant
*CARDAMOM *Eletaria cardamomum* *Zingiberaceae*	pungent, sweet	heating	pungent	VK – P+	stimulant, carminative, expectorant
CASCARA SAGRADA *Rhamnus purshianus* *Rhamnaceae*	bitter	cooling	pungent	PK – V+	laxative, astringent, bitter, tonic
CASTOR OIL *Ricinus communis* *Euphorbiaceae*	pungent, sweet	heating	pungent	V – PK+	carthartic, demulcent, analgesic, nervine

Herb	Taste	Energy	Post-digestive	Effect	Actions
CATNIP *Nepeta cataria* Labiatae	pungent	cooling	pungent	PK– Vo	diaphoretic, carminative, nervine
CATTAIL *Typha spp.* Typhaceae	sweet, astringent	cooling	sweet	P– VK+	astringent, hemostatic, vulnerary
CAYENNE *Capsicum annuum* Solanaceae	pungent	heating	pungent	KV– P+	stimulant, carminative, alterative, hemostatic
CENTAURY, AMERICAN *Sabbatia angularis* Gentianaceae	bitter	cooling	pungent	PK– V+	febrifuge, bitter tonic
CENTAURY, EUROPEAN *Erythraea centaurium* Gentianaceae	bitter, pungent	cooling	pungent	PK– V+	bitter tonic, antipyretic
CHAMOMILE *Matricaria chamomilla (Ger.)* *Anthemis nobilis (Roman)* Compositae	bitter, pungent	cooling	pungent	PK– Vo	diaphoretic, carminative, nervine
CHAPARRAL *Larrea divaricata* Zygophyllaceae	bitter	cooling	pungent	PK– V+	alterative, diuretic, bitter tonic
CHIA SEEDS *Salvia polystachya* Labiatae	pungent, sweet	heating	sweet	KV– P+	expectorant, demulcent, diaphoretic

HERB	TASTE	ENERGY	PD-EFFECT	DOSHA	ACTIONS
CHICKWEED *Stellaria media* Caryophyllaceae	bitter, sweet	cooling	sweet	PK – V+	alterative, demulcent, laxative, vulnerary
CHICORY *Cichorium intybus* Compositae	bitter	cooling	pungent	PK – V+	alterative, diuretic, antipyretic
CILANTRO *Coriandrum sativum* Umbelliferae	bitter, pungent	cooling	pungent	PK – Vo	alterative, carminative, diuretic
*CINNAMON *Cinnamomum Zeylanicum, etc.* Lauraceae	pungent, sweet astringent	heating	sweet	VK – P+	stimulant, diaphoretic, alterative
CLEAVERS *Galium aparine* Rubiaceae	astringent, bitter	cooling	pungent	PK – V+	diuretic, alterative, vulnerary
*CLOVES *Eugenia caryophyllata* Myrtaceae	pungent	heating	pungent	VK – P+	stimulant, carminative, aphrodisiac, expectorant
COCONUT *Cocus nucifera* Palmae	sweet	cooling	sweet	PV – K+	refrigerant, diuretic, tonic
COLTSFOOT *Tussilago farfara* Compositae	pungent, astringent, sweet	cooling	pungent	PK – Vo	demulcent, expectorant, astringent, antispasmodic

*COMFREY *Symphytum officinale* Boraginaceae	sweet, astringent	cooling	sweet	PV– K+	nutritive tonic, demulcent, emollient, vulnerary
*CORIANDER *Coriandrum sativum* Umbelliferae	bitter, pungent	cooling	pungent	PKV=	alterative, diaphoretic, diuretic, carminative
CORN SILK *Zea mays* Graminaceae	sweet	cooling	pungent	PK– V+	diuretic, demulcent, alterative
COTTON ROOT *Gossypium herbaceum* Malvaceae	sweet	heating	sweet	V– KP+	nutritive tonic, aphrodisiac, emmenagogue
CRAMPBARK *Viburnum opulus* Caprifoliaceae	bitter, astringent	heating	pungent	KV– P+	emmenagogue, astringent, antispasmodic
CRANESBILL *Geranium maculatum* Geraniaceae	astringent	cooling	pungent	PK– V+	astringent, hemostatic, vulnerary
CUBEBS *Piper cubeba* Piperaceae	pungent	heating	pungent	VK– P+	stimulant, carminative, expectorant
CULVER'S ROOT *Leptandra virginica* Scrophulariaceae	bitter	cooling	pungent	PK– V+	cathartic, febrifuge, bitter tonic

HERB	TASTE	ENERGY	PD-EFFECT	DOSHA	ACTIONS
CUMIN *Cuminum cyminum* *Umbelliferae*	pungent, bitter	cooling	pungent	PKV =	carminative, alterative, stimulant
DAMIANA *Turnera aphrodisiaca* *Turneraceae*	pungent, bitter	heating	pungent	K – Vo P+	stimulant, aphrodisiac
***DANDELION** *Taraxacum officinalis* *Compositae*	bitter, sweet	cooling	pungent	PK – V+	alterative, diuretic, laxative
DATES *Phoenix dacytlifera* *Palmae*	sweet	cooling	sweet	VP – K+	demulcent, tonic, aphrodisiac
DEVIL'S CLAW *Harpagophytum procumbens* *Pedaliaceae*	bitter, astringent	cooling	pungent	PK – V+	alterative, anti-inflammatory, analgesic
DILL *Anethum graveolens* *Umbelliferae*	pungent, bitter	cooling	pungent	PK – Vo	carminative, alterative, expectorant
***ECHINACEA** *Echinacea augustifolia* *Compositae*	bitter, pungent	cooling	pungent	PK – V+	alterative, antibiotic, diaphoretic

Herb					
ELDER FLOWERS *Sambucus spp.* *Caprifoliaceae*	bitter, pungent	cooling	pungent	KP– Vo	diaphoretic, diuretic, alterative
***ELECAMPANE** *Inula spp.* *Compositae*	pungent, bitter	heating	pungent	VK– P+	expectorant, antispasmodic, rejuvenative
ELEUTHRO *Eleuthro senticosus* *Araliaceae*	pungent, sweet	heating	sweet	VK– P+	tonic, antispasmodic, antirheumatic
EUCALYPTUS *Eucalyptus globulus* *Myrtaceae*	pungent	heating	pungent	KV– P+	diaphoretic, decongestant, stimulant
EYEBRIGHT *Euphrasia officinalis* *Scrophulariaceae*	bitter	cooling	pungent	PK– V+	antipyretic, alterative, astringent
FALSE UNICORN *Helonias dioica* *Liliaceae*	bitter, sweet	heating	sweet	VK– P+	emmenagogue, aphrodisiac, diuretic
***FENNEL** *Foeniculum vulgare* *Umbelliferae*	sweet, pungent	cooling	sweet	VPK=	carminative, diuretic, antispasmodic
***FENUGREEK** *Trigonella foenumgraecum* *Leguminosae*	bitter, pungent sweet	heating	pungent	VK– P+	stimulant, tonic, expectorant, rejuvenative

HERB	TASTE	ENERGY	PD-EFFECT	DOSHA	ACTIONS
*FLAXSEED *Linum usitatissimum* *Linaceae*	sweet, astringent	heating	pungent	V– Ko P+	laxative, demulcent, nutritive tonic
FRANKINCENSE *Boswellia thurifera* *Burseraceae*	bitter, pungent astringent, sweet	heating	pungent	KV – P+	alterative, analgesic, rejuvenative
GALANGAL *Alpinia officinarum* *Zingiberaceae*	pungent	heating	pungent	VK – P+	stimulant, diaphoretic, antirheumatic
*GARLIC *Allium sativum* *Liliaceae*	all but sour	heating	pungent	VK – P+	stimulant, carminative, expectorant, alterative
*GENTIAN *Gentiana spp.* *Liliaceae*	bitter	cooling	pungent	PK – V+	bitter tonic, antipyretic, alterative
*GINGER *Zingiber officinale* *Zingiberaceae*	pungent, sweet	heating	sweet	VK – P+	stimulant, diaphoretic, expectorant, carminative
GOLD THREAD *Coptis spp.* *Ranunculaceae*	bitter	cooling	pungent	PK – V+	bitter tonic, antipyretic, alterative

Herb	Rasa	Virya	Vipaka	Dosha	Actions
*GOLDEN SEAL *Hydrastis canadensis* *Ranunculaceae*	bitter, astringent	cooling	pungent	PK– V+	bitter tonic, antipyretic antibiotic
GRAPES (Raisins) *Vitis vinifera* *Vitaceae*	sweet	cooling	sweet	PV– K+	nutritive tonic, demulcent, laxative
GRAVEL ROOT *Eupatorium purpureum* *Compositae*	bitter, pungent	cooling	pungent	PK– V+	diuretic, lithotriptic, nervine
GRINDELIA *Grindelia spp.* *Compositae*	pungent	heating	pungent	KV– P+	expectorant, diaphoretic, antispasmodic
GROUND IVY *Glechoma hederacea* *Labiatae*	pungent, astringent	heating	pungent	KV– P+	diaphoretic, astringent, carminative
GUM ARABIC *Acacia senegal* *Leguminosae*	sweet	cooling	sweet	PV– K+	demulcent, emollient, tonic
*HAWTHORN *Crataegus oxycantha* *Rosaceae*	sour, sweet	heating	sour	V–Ko P+	stimulant, antispasmodic, diuretic
HENNA *Lawsonia spp.* *Lythraceae*	bitter, astringent	cooling	pungent	PK– V+	antipyretic, alterative, nervine

HERB	TASTE	ENERGY	PD-EFFECT	DOSHA	ACTIONS
*HIBISCUS *Hibiscus rosa-sinensis* *Malvaceae*	astringent, sweet	cooling	sweet	PK – V+	alterative, hemostatic, refrigerant, emmenagogue
HONEY	sweet, pungent, astringent	heating	sweet	VK – P+	expectorant, emollient, tonic, laxative
HOPS *Humulus lupulus* *Articaceae*	bitter, pungent	cooling	pungent	PK – V+	nervine, bitter tonic, diuretic
HOREHOUND *Marrubium vulgare* *Labiatae*	bitter, pungent	cooling	pungent	KP – V+	expectorant, antispasmodic, diaphoretic
HORSERADISH *Cochlearia armoracia* *Cruciferae*	pungent	heating	pungent	KV – P+	stimulant, diuretic, carminative
*HORSETAIL *Equisetum spp.* *Equisetaceae*	bitter, sweet	cooling	pungent	PK – V+	diuretic, diaphoretic, alterative
HYSSOP *Hyssopus officinalis* *Labiatae*	pungent, bitter	heating	pungent	KV – P+	diaphoretic, diuretic, carminative, anthelmintic
ICELAND MOSS *Cetraria islandica* *Algae*	salty, sweet, astringent	cooling	sweet	PV – K+	demulcent, alterative, tonic

INDIGO *Indigofera tinctoria* *Leguminosae*	bitter	cooling	pungent	PK– V+	alterative, antibiotic, laxative
*IRISH MOSS *Chondrus crispus* *Algae*	salty, sweet, astringent	heating	sweet	V – PK+	nutritive tonic, demulcent, emollient
*JUNIPER BERRIES *Juniperus spp.* *Coniferae*	pungent, bitter, sweet	heating	pungent	KV – P +	diuretic, diaphoretic, carminative, analgesic
KELP *Fucus visiculosis*	salty, sweet	heating	sweet	V – KP+	nutritive tonic, demulcent, expectorant
KUDZU *Pueraria tuberosa* *Leguminosae*	sweet	cooling	sweet	PV – K+	tonic, diaphoretic, diuretic
LADY'S SLIPPER *Cypripedium pubescens* *Orchidaceae*	pungent, sweet, bitter	heating	sweet	VK – Po	nervine, antispasmodic, tonic
LAVENDER *Lavandula spp.* *Labiatae*	pungent	cooling	pungent	PK– Vo	carminative, diuretic, antispasmodic
LEMON *Citrus limonum* *Rutaceae*	sour	cooling	sour	PV – Ko	expectorant, carminative, astringent

HERB	TASTE	ENERGY	PD-EFFECT	DOSHA	ACTIONS
LEMON BALM *Melissa officinalis* *Labiatae*	pungent, sweet	cooling	pungent	KP– Vo	diaphoretic, carminative, nervine
LEMON GRASS *Cymbopogon citratus* *Graminaceae*	pungent, bitter	cooling	pungent	PK– Vo	diuretic, diaphoretic, refrigerant
*LICORICE *Glycyrrhiza glabra* *Leguminosae*	sweet, bitter	cooling	sweet	VP– K+	demulcent, expectorant, tonic, laxative
LILY *Lilium spp.* *Liliceae*	sweet	cooling	sweet	VP– K+	demulcent, nutritive tonic, nervine
LIME *Citrus acida* *Rutaceae*	sour, bitter	cooling	sour	PV– K+	refrigerant, carminative, expectorant
LOBELIA *Lobelia inflata* *Lobeliaceae*	pungent	heating	pungent	K– PV+	antispasmodic, emetic, expectorant, diaphoretic
MACE *Myristica fragrans* *Myristicaceae*	pungent, sweet	heating	pungent	VK– P+	antispasmodic, emetic, expectorant, diaphoretic

Herb					
MAIDENHAIR FERN *Adiandum capillus-veneris* *Filices*	sweet, bitter	cooling	sweet	PV– K+	demulcent, refrigerant, tonic
MALE FERN *Dryopteris filix-mas* *Filices*	bitter, pungent	cooling	pungent	PK– V+	anthelmintic
MALVA *Malva spp.* *Malvaceae*	sweet, astringent	cooling	sweet	PV– K+	demulcent, emollient, astringent
MANDRAKE, AMERICAN *Podophyllum peltatum* *Berberidaceae*	bitter	cooling	pungent	PK– V+	cathartic, alterative, toxic
MARJORAM *Origanum marjorana* *Labiatae*	pungent	heating	pungent	VK– P+	stimulant, antispasmodic, diaphoretic
*MARSHMALLOW *Althea officinalis* *Malvaceae*	sweet	cooling	sweet	PV– K+	tonic, demulcent, diuretic, laxative
MISTLETOE *Viscum album* *Loranthaceae*	bitter, sweet	heating	pungent	VK– P+	nervine, antispasmodic, emmenagogue
MORMON TEA *Ephedra spp.* *Gnetaceae*	pungent	heating	pungent	K– VP+	diuretic, alterative

HERB	TASTE	ENERGY	PD-EFFECT	DOSHA	ACTIONS
MOTHERWORT *Leonurus cardiaca* *Labiatae*	bitter, pungent	cooling	pungent	PK– V+	emmenagogue, diaphoretic, diuretic, alterative
***MUGWORT** *Artemesia vulgaris* *Compositae*	pungent, bitter	heating	pungent	VK– P+	antispasmodic, diaphoretic, emmenagogue
***MULLEIN** *Verbascum thapsus* *Scrophulariaceae*	bitter, astringent, sweet	cooling	pungent	PK– V+	expectorant, astringent, vulnerary, sedative
MUSTARD SEEDS *Brassica alba* *Cruciferae*	pungent	heating	pungent	KV– P+	stimulant, expectorant, carminative
***MYRRH** *Commiphora myrrha* *Burseraceae*	bitter, pungent	heating	pungent	KV– P+	alterative, analgesic, emmenagogue, rejuvenative
NETTLE *Urtica urens* *Urticaceae*	astringent	cooling	pungent	PK– V+	alterative, astringent, hemostatic
***NUTMEG** *Myristica fragrans* *Myristicaceae*	pungent	heating	pungent	VK– P+	astringent, carminative, sedative, nervine
OAT STRAW *Avena sativa* *Graminaceae*	sweet	cooling	sweet	VP– K+	nervine, antispasmodic, tonic

Herb					
ONION *Allium cepa* *Liliaceae*	pungent, sweet	heating	sweet	VK– P+	diaphoretic, tonic, aphrodisiac
ORANGE PEEL *Citrus aurantium* *Rutaceae*	pungent, bitter	heating	pungent	VK– P+	carminative, expectorant, stimulant
OREGANO *Origanum vulgare* *Labiatae*	pungent	heating	pungent	VK– P+	stimulant, carminative, diaphoretic
OREGON GRAPE *Mahonia repens* *Berberidaceae*	bitter	heating	pungent	PK– V+	alterative, antipyretic, laxative
OSHA *Ligusticum porteri* *Umbelliferae*	pungent, bitter	heating	pungent	KV– P+	stimulant, antibacterial, expectorant
PAPRIKA *Capsicum annuum* *Solanaceae*	pungent	heating	pungent	KV– P+	stimulant, carminative
*PARSLEY *Petroselinum spp.* *Umbelliferae*	pungent	heating	pungent	KV– P+	diuretic, emmenagogue, carminative
PASSION FLOWER *Passiflora incarnata* *Passifloraceae*	bitter	cooling	pungent	PK– V+	nervine, sedative, diuretic, anodyne

HERB	TASTE	ENERGY	PD-EFFECT	DOSHA	ACTIONS
PAU D'ARCO *Tabebuia avellanedae* *Bignoneaceae*	bitter	cooling	pungent	PK– V+	alterative, antipyretic, antibiotic
***PENNYROYAL** *Mentha pulegium* *Labiatae*	pungent	heating	pungent	VK– P+	diaphoretic, carminative, emmenagogue
PEONY *Paeonia officinalis* *Ranunculaceae*	bitter, astringent	cooling	sweet	PK– Vo	alterative, emmenagogue, nervine
***PEPPERMINT** *Mentha piperita* *Labiatae*	pungent	cooling	pungent	PK– Vo	diaphoretic, carminative, nervine
PERUVIAN BARK *Cinchona succirubra* *Rubiaceae*	bitter	cooling	pungent	PK– V+	bitter tonic, antipyretic
PIPSISSEWA *Chimaphila umbellata* *Ericaceae*	bitter	cooling	pungent	PK– V+	diuretic, astringent, alterative
PLANTAIN *Plantago major* *Plantaginaceae*	astringent, bitter	cooling	pungent	PK– V+	astringent, alterative, diuretic, vulnerary
PLEURISY ROOT *Asclepias tuberosa* *Asclepiadaceae*	bitter, pungent	cooling	pungent	PK– V+	diaphoretic, expectorant, febrifuge

Name	Taste	Energy	Post-digestive	Dosha	Actions
POKEROOT *Phytolacca spp.* *Phytolaccaceae*	bitter	cooling	pungent	PK– V+	alterative, emetic, cathartic
***POMEGRANATE** *Punica granatum* *Lythraceae*	astringent, bitter, sweet	cooling	sweet	PK– Vo	astringent, alterative, anthelmintic, tonic
***POPPY SEEDS** *Papaver spp.* *Papaveraceae*	pungent, astringent, sweet	heating	sweet	VK– P+	astringent, carminative, sedative
***PRICKLY ASH** *Xanthoxylum spp.* *Rutaceae*	pungent, bitter	heating	pungent	VK– P+	stimulant, carminative, anthelmintic
PRIMROSE *Primula vulgaris* *Primulaceae*	bitter	cooling	pungent	PK– V+	nervine, alterative, expectorant
***PSYLLIUM** *Plantago psyllium* *Plantaginaceae*	sweet, astringent	cooling	sweet	PV– K+	laxative, demulcent, astringent
PUMPKIN SEEDS *Cucurbita pepo* *Cucurbiaceae*	sweet	heating	sweet	V– PK+	anthelmintic, diuretic
PURPLE LOOSESTRIFE *Lythrum salicaria* *Lythraceae*	astringent, sweet	cooling	pungent	PK– V+	alterative, astringent, demulcent

HERB	TASTE	ENERGY	PD-EFFECT	DOSHA	ACTIONS
*RASPBERRY *Rubus spp.* *Rosaceae*	astringent, sweet	cooling	sweet	PK– V+	astringent, alterative, emmenagogue
*RED CLOVER *Trifolium pratense* *Leguminosae*	bitter, sweet	cooling	pungent	PK– V+	alterative, diuretic, expectorant
RED ROOT *Ceanothus spp.* *Rhamnaceae*	astringent	cooling	pungent	PK– V+	astringent, expectorant, sedative
*RHUBARB *Rheum spp.* *Polygonaceae*	bitter	cooling	pungent	PK– V+	purgative, alterative, antipyretic
*ROSE FLOWERS *Rosa spp.* *Rosaceae*	bitter, pungent, astringent, sweet	cooling	sweet	VPK=	alterative, emmenagogue, nervine
ROSE HIPS *Rosa spp.* *Rosaceae*	sour, astringent	heating	sour	V– KP+	stimulant, carminative, astringent
ROSEMARY *Rosmarinus officinalis* *Labiatae*	pungent, bitter	heating	pungent	KV– P+	diaphoretic, carminative, stimulant, emmenagogue

RUE *Ruta graveolens* *Rutaceae*	bitter, pungent	heating	pungent	KV – P+	nervine, emmenagogue, anthelmintic
SAFFLOWER *Carthamus tinctorius* *Compositae*	pungent	heating	pungent	VK – P+	alterative, emmenagogue, carminative
*****SAFFRON** *Crocus sativus* *Iridaceae*	pungent, bitter, sweet	cooling	sweet	VPK=	alterative, emmenagogue, rejuvenative, carminative
*****SAGE** *Salvia officinalis* *Labiatae*	pungent, bitter, astringent	heating	pungent	KV – P+	diaphoretic, expectorant, nervine, astringent
*****SANDALWOOD** *Santalum album* *Santalaceae*	bitter, sweet, astringent	cooling	sweet	PV – Ko	alterative, hemostatic, antipyretic, nervine
*****SARSAPARILLA** *Smilax spp.* *Liliaceae*	bitter, sweet	cooling	sweet	PV – Ko	alterative, diuretic, antispasmodic
SASSAFRAS *Sassafras officinale* *lauraceae*	pungent	heating	pungent	KV – P+	alterative, diaphoretic, stimulant
SAVORY *Satureia hortensis* *Labiatae*	pungent	heating	pungent	KV – P+	stimulant, carminative, astringent

HERB	TASTE	ENERGY	PD-EFFECT	DOSHA	ACTIONS
SAW PALMETTO *Serenoa serrulata* *Palmaceae*	sweet, pungent	heating	sweet	V – PK+	tonic, rejuvenative, aphrodisiac, expectorant
SELF-HEAL *Prunella vulgaris* *Labiatae*	bitter, astringent	cooling	pungent	PK – V+	alterative, antipyretic, vulnerary
*SENNA *Cassia acutifolia* *Leguminosae*	bitter	cooling	pungent	PK – V+	purgative, antipyretic, alterative
*SESAME SEEDS *Sesamum indicum* *Pedaliaceae*	sweet	heating	sweet	V – PK+	nutritive tonic, demulcent, rejuvenative
SHEPHERD'S PURSE *Capsella bursapastoris* *Cruciferae*	astringent, bitter	cooling	pungent	PK – V+	astringent, hemostatic, alterative
*SKULLCAP *Scutellaria spp.* *Labiatae*	bitter	cooling	pungent	PK – Vo	nervine, antispasmodic
SKUNK CABBAGE *Symplocarpus foetidus* *Araceae*	pungent	heating	pungent	KV – P+	nervine, antispasmodic, expectorant
*SLIPPERY ELM *Ulmus fulva* *Urticaceae*	sweet	cooling	sweet	PV – K+	nutritive tonic, demulcent, emollient

Herb	Taste	Energy	Post-digestive	Dosha	Actions
*SOLOMON'S SEAL *Polygonatum spp.* *Liliaceae*	sweet, bitter	cooling	sweet	PV– K+	nutritive tonic, demulcent, astringent, rejuvenative
*SPEARMINT *Mentha spicata* *Labiatae*	pungent	cooling	pungent	KP– Vo	diaphoretic, diuretic, carminative
SPIKENARD *Aralia racemosa* *Araliaceae*	sweet, pungent	heating	sweet	KV– P+	demulcent, expectorant, tonic, alterative
SQUAW VINE *Mitchella repens* *Rubiaceae*	astringent, bitter	cooling	pungent	PK– V+	emmenagogue, astringent, diuretic, alterative
ST. JOHN'S WORT *Hypericum perforatum* *Hypericaceae*	bitter, pungent	cooling	pungent	PK– V+	antispasmodic, expectorant, astringent
STAR ANISE *Illicium verum* *Magnoliaceae*	pungent	heating	pungent	VK– P+	stimulant, carminative
STILLINGIA *Stillingia sylvatica* *Euphorbiaceae*	pungent	heating	pungent	KV– P+	alterative, diaphoretic, expectorant, tonic
STONEROOT *Collinsonia canadensis* *Labiatae*	bitter	cooling	pungent	PK– V+	diuretic, diaphoretic, astringent

HERB	TASTE	ENERGY	PD-EFFECT	DOSHA	ACTIONS
STRAWBERRY LEAVES *Fragaria spp.* *Rosaceae*	astringent, sweet	cooling	sweet	PK – V+	alterative, astringent, diuretic
SUGAR *Saccharum officinarum* *Graminae*	sweet	cooling	sweet	PV – K+	nutritive tonic, demulcent, laxative
SUMACH *Rhus glabra, etc.* *Anacardiaceae*	astringent	cooling	pungent	PK – V+	astringent, alterative, refrigerant
TAMARIND *Tamarindus indica* *Leguminosae*	sour, sweet	heating	sour	VK – P+	stimulant, carminative, laxative
TANSY *Tanacetum vulgare* *Compositae*	bitter, pungent	cooling	pungent	PK – Vo	emmenagogue, diaphoretic, bitter tonic
TARRAGON *Artemesia dracunculus* *Compositae*	bitter, pungent	heating	pungent	KV – P+	emmenagogue, diuretic, carminative
THYME *Thymus vulgaris* *Labiatae*	pungent	heating	pungent	VK – P+	antispasmodic, carminative, antispasmodic

Herb	Taste	Energy	Vipaka	Dosha	Actions
TORMENTIL *Potentilla tormentilla* Rosaceae	astringent, bitter	cooling	pungent	PK– V+	astringent, hemostatic, antiseptic
*TURMERIC *Curcuma longa* Zingiberaceae	pungent, bitter,	heating	pungent	KV– Po	stimulant, alterative, antibacterial, vulnerary
UVA URSI *Arctostaphylos uva-ursi* Ericaceae	astringent, bitter	cooling	pungent	PK– V+	diuretic, astringent, antiseptic
*VALERIAN *Valeriana spp.* Valerianaceae	pungent	heating	pungent	VK– P+	nervine, antispasmodic, carminative, sedative
VERVAIN *Verbena spp.* Verbenaceae	bitter	cooling	pungent	PK– V+	antipyretic, expectorant, astringent
VETIVERIAN *Andropogon muricatus* Graminaceae	bitter, sweet	cooling	pungent	PK– V+	antipyretic, astringent refrigerant
VIOLET *Viola spp.* Violaceae	bitter, pungent	cooling	pungent	PK– V+	alterative, antiseptic, expectorant
WAHOO *Euonymus atropurpureus* Celastraceae	bitter	cooling	pungent	PK– V+	purgative, antipyretic, diuretic

HERB	TASTE	ENERGY	PD-EFFECT	DOSHA	ACTIONS
WALNUT *Juglans nigra* Juglandaceae	sweet	heating	sweet	V – PK+	demulcent, tonic, laxative
WATERCRESS *Rorippa nasturtium* Cruciferae	pungent	heating	pungent	KV – P+	diuretic, expectorant, stimulant
WHITE OAK *Quercus alba* Cupuliferae	astringent	cooling	pungent	PK – V+	astringent, hemostatic, antiseptic
WHITE PINE *Pinus alba* Pinaceae	pungent	heating	pungent	KV – P+	expectorant, diaphoretic, carminative
*WHITE POND LILY *Nymphaea odorata* Nymphaeaceae	sweet, astringent, bitter	cooling	sweet	PV – K+	demulcent, astringent, tonic
WHITE POPLAR *Populus tremuloides* Salicaceae	bitter	cooling	pungent	PK – V+	bitter tonic, antipyretic, diuretic
WILD CARROT *Daucus carota* Umbelliferae	pungent	heating	pungent	KV – P+	diuretic, stimulant, carminative, emmenagogue
*WILD CHERRY BARK *Prunus spp.* Rosaceae	bitter, astringent	cooling	sweet	PK – Vo	antispasmodic, expectorant, alterative

Herb	Taste	Energy		Dosha	Actions
WILD GINGER *Asarum Canadense* *Aristolochiaceae*	pungent	heating	pungent	KV– P+	diaphoretic, expectorant, decongestant
WILLOW BARK *Salix spp.* *Salicaceae*	bitter	cooling	pungent	PK– V+	bitter tonic, antipyretic, anodyne
WINTERGREEN *Gaultheria procumbens* *Ericaceae*	pungent	cooling	pungent	PK– Vo	carminative, astringent, analgesic
WITCH HAZEL *Hamamelis virginiana* *Hamamelidaceae*	astringent, bitter, pungent	cooling	pungent	PK– V+	astringent, hemostatic, vulnerary
WORMSEED *Chenopodium anthelminticum* *Chenopodiaceae*	pungent, bitter, astringent	heating	pungent	KV– P+	anthelmintic, stimulant, antispasmodic
WORMWOOD *Artemisia absinthium* *Compositae*	bitter, pungent, astringent	cooling	pungent	PK– Vo	anthelmintic, carminative, antispasmodic
*YARROW *Achillea millefolium* *Compositae*	bitter, pungent astringent	cooling	pungent	PK– V+	diaphoretic, astringent, alterative
*YELLOW DOCK *Rumex crispus* *Polygonaceae*	bitter, astringent	cooling	pungent	PK– V+	alterative, astringent, laxative

HERB	TASTE	ENERGY	PD-EFFECT	DOSHA	ACTIONS
YERBA SANTA *Eriodictyon glutinosum* *Hydrophyllaceae*	pungent	heating	pungent	KV– P+	expectorant, antispasmodic, carminative
YERBA MATÉ *Ilex paraguariensis* *Aquifoliaceae*	pungent	heating	pungent	K– Vo P+	stimulant, diuretic
SPECIAL HERBS					
***AJWAN** *Apium graveolens* *Umbelliferae*	pungent	heating	pungent	KV– P+	stimulant, diaphoretic, antispasmodic
***AMALAKI** *Emblica officinalis* *Euphorbiaceae*	all but salty	cooling	sweet	PV– Ko	nutritive tonic, rejuvenative, alterative
***ANGELICA(Tang kuei)** *Angelica spp.* *Umbelliferae*	pungent, sweet	heating	sweet	VK– Po	tonic, emmenagogue, rejuvenative, diaphoretic
***ASAFOETIDA** *Ferula asafoetida* *Umbelliferae*	pungent	heating	pungent	VK– P+	stimulant, carminative, antispasmodic, anthelmintic
***ASHWAGANDHA** *Withania somnifera* *Solanaceae*	bitter, astringent	heating	sweet	VK– P+	tonic, rejuvenative, aphrodisiac, nervine

Herb	Rasa (taste)	Virya (energy)	Vipaka	Dosha	Actions
ATIBALA *Abutilon indicum* Malvaceae	sweet	cooling	sweet	PK–Vo	tonic, demulcent, diuretic, laxative
*BALA *Sida cordifolia* Malvaceae	sweet	cooling	sweet	VP–Ko	tonic, nervine, demulcent, rejuvenative
*BHRINGARAJ *Eclipta alba, etc.* Compositae	bitter, astringent, sweet	cooling	sweet	VPK=	tonic, alterative, nervine, hemostatic
*BIBHITAKI *Terminalia belerica* Combretaceae	astringent	heating	sweet	KP–Vo	tonic, astringent, expectorant, laxative
*CHRYSANTHEMUM *Chrysanthemum indicum* Compositae	bitter, sweet	cooling	pungent	PK–V+	diaphoretic, antipyretic, alterative
*EPHEDRA *Ephedra vulgaris* Gnetaceae	pungent	heating	pungent	K–VP+	diaphoretic, diuretic, anti-cough, stimulant
*FO-TI *Polygonum multiflorum* Polygonaceae	sweet, bitter, astringent	cooling	sweet	PV–K+	tonic, rejuvenative, aphrodisiac, astringent
*GINSENG *Panax ginseng* Araliaceae	pungent, bitter, sweet	heating	sweet	V–KPo	tonic, stimulant, rejuvenative

HERB	TASTE	ENERGY	PD-EFFECT	DOSHA	ACTIONS
*GOKSHURA *Tribulis terrestris* Zygophyllaceae	sweet, bitter	cooling	sweet	PK – Vo	diuretic, tonic, aphrodisiac
*GOTU KOLA *Hydrocotyle asiatica* Umbelliferae	bitter	cooling	sweet	PKV =	nervine, rejuvenative, alterative, diuretic
*GUGGUL *Commiphora mukul* Burseaceae	bitter, pungent, astringent, sweet	heating	pungent	KV – P+	rejuvenative, alterative, antispasmodic, expectorant
*HARITAKI *Terminalia chebula* Combretaceae	all but salty	heating	sweet	VK – Po	rejuvenative, nervine, astringent, laxative
*JASMINE FLOWERS *Jasminum grandiflorum* Oleaceae	bitter	cooling	pungent	PK – V+	alterative, refrigerant, emmenagogue, nervine
*LOTUS *Nelumbo nucifera* Nymphaeaceae	sweet, astringent	cooling	sweet	PV – K+	nutritive tonic, aphrodisiac, astringent, nervine
MAHABALA *Sida rhombifolia* Malvaceae	sweet, bitter	cooling	sweet	PV – Ko	tonic, demulcent, rejuvenative, diuretic
*MANJISHTA *Rubia cordifolia* Rubiaceae	bitter, sweet	cooling	pungent	PK – V+	alterative, hemostatic, emmenagogue, diuretic

*MUSTA *Cyperus rotundus* Cyperaceae	pungent, bitter	cooling	pungent	PK– V o	carminative, astringent, alterative, emmenagogue
*NEEM *Azadiracta indica* Meliaceae	bitter	cooling	pungent	PK– V+	bitter tonic, antipyretic, alterative
*PIPPALI *Piper longum* Piperaceae	pungent	heating	sweet	VK– P+	stimulant, expectorant, aphrodisiac
*PUNARNAVA *Boerhaavia diffusa* Nyctagineae	bitter	cooling	pungent	PK– V+	diuretic, diaphoretic, laxative, rejuvenative
*REHMANNIA *Rehmannia glutinosa* Scrophulariaceae	sweet, bitter	cooling	sweet	PV– K+	nutritive tonic, rejuvenative, aphrodisiac
*SHATAVARI *Asparagus racemosus* Liliaceae	sweet, bitter	cooling	sweet	PV– K+	nutritive tonic, demulcent, emmenagogue, rejuvenative
*VAMSHA ROCHANA *Bambusa arundinaceae* Gramineae	sweet, astringent	cooling	sweet	PV– K+	demulcent, expectorant, tonic
*VIDARI-KANDA *Ipomoea digitata* Convolvulaceae	sweet	cooling	sweet	VP– K o	nutritive tonic, aphrodisiac, diuretic
*WILD YAM *Dioscorea spp.* Dioscoreaceae	sweet, bitter	cooling	sweet	VP– K o	antispasmodic, diaphoretic, tonic, rejuvenative

APPENDIX III

FIRST AID TREATMENTS

Acne: Apply a turmeric and sandalwood powder paste externally using ½ tsp. of each and adding sufficient water to make a paste. One may also take 1 tbs. of aloe vera gel internally with ¼ tsp. turmeric 2 times per day until the acne clears.

Asthma: Elecampane root tea is effective, to which can be added ½ part each of ginger and licorice, 1-2 tsp. of herbs per cup of boiling water; or equal parts thyme and comfrey root can be used in a similar manner. For severe asthmatic attacks consult a medical practitioner.

Backache: Apply ginger paste and then eucalyptus oil to the affected area.

Bad breath: Cleanse the mouth with licorice powder and chew fennel seeds. For internal usage make an infusion of cardamom, cinnamon and bay leaves, equal parts, 1 tsp. per cup.

Bleeding (external): Apply ice or a sandalwood paste. The black ash of a burned cotton ball may also be applied to the site of external bleeding or a poultice of comfrey leaves or yarrow.

Bleeding (internal): Drink a cup of warm milk to which has been added ½ tsp. of turmeric and a pinch of saffron or alum.

Boils: To bring a skin boil to a head, apply cooked onions as a poultice or apply a paste of ginger powder and turmeric (½ tsp. of each) directly to the boil.

Burns: Make a paste of fresh gel of aloe vera with a pinch of turmeric powder. *Ghee* or coconut oil also may be used.

Common Cold: Take 1 tbs. grated fresh ginger with 1 tsp. cinnamon and 1 tsp. licorice and boil in 1 quart of water for 10 minutes. Take 1 cup every 3 hours sweetened with a little honey. Or simply take fresh ginger tea.

Constipation: Severe: Take an infusion of rhubarb root (1 tsp. per cup), along with ¼ tsp. each ginger powder and licorice (increase dosage if necessary). Moderate: Take 1-2 tsps. of Psyllium husk powder in a cup of warm water before sleep. Mild: Take 1 tsp. of *ghee* in a cup of warm milk.

Cough: Drink elecampane root tea, to which smaller amounts of ginger and licorice can be added, 1-2 tsp. of the herbs per cup of boiling water; sweeten with honey. For mucus, prepare a tea of ½ tsp. ginger powder, cloves and cinnamon ¼ tsp. each, per cup; sweeten with honey.

Dehydration: To 1 pint of distilled water, add ¼ tsp. of salt plus 3 tsps. of natural raw cane sugar. Add 2 tsps. lime juice. Mix, and sip orally.

Diarrhea: Blend together ½ cup yogurt and ½ cup water to which 1 tsp. grated fresh ginger has been added and a little nutmeg. For dysentery, take equal parts barberry and raspberry leaves along with ½ part nutmeg. Make an infusion 2-3 tsps. per cup and take every few hours until condition improves.

Earache: Place 3 drops of garlic oil in the ear; or use a mixture of 1 tsp. of onion juice with ½ tsp. of honey and introduce 5 to 10 drops into the ear.

Ear ringing: Put 3 drops of clove oil into the ear.

Exhaustion (heat): Apply sandalwood oil to the forehead or drink sandalwood tea. Drink coconut water or grape juice.

Eyes (burning): Apply several drops of pure rose water or fresh aloe vera gel into the affected eye. Internally, chrysanthemum or chamomile tea may be taken (1-2 tsp. per cup).

Food Poisoning/Radiation: In 1 cup of miso soup, add 1 tsp. of *ghee* and ½ tsp. each of coriander and cumin powder.

Gas (abdominal): Make an infusion of cardamom, fennel and ginger, equal parts, 1 tsp. per cup of water, to which a pinch of asafoetida may be added.

Gums (bleeding): Apply powdered myrrh to the gums or drink lemon juice. The gums may be massaged with coconut oil.

Headaches: For general relief of headaches, a paste of ½ tsp. of ginger powder, mixed with water and heated, is applied to the forehead. A burning sensation may possibly occur but it will not be harmful.

The following can be useful for relief of specific types of headaches. Sinus headaches relate to *kapha* and can be relieved by applying a ginger paste to the forehead and sinuses. Temporal headaches indicate an excess of *pitta* in the stomach. They can be relieved by drinking a tea of cumin and coriander seeds, ½ tsp. of each in one cup of hot water. At the same time, apply sandalwood oil or a sandalwood paste to the temples. Occipital headaches indicate toxins in the colon. Take 2 tsps. of flaxseed before sleep in one cup of warm milk. At the same time, apply a ginger paste behind the ears (mastoid processes).

Hemorrhoids: Drink ½ tbs. of aloe vera gel with a little ginger twice a day until hemorrhoids disappear.

Hiccups: Take 2 parts honey with 1 part castor oil, 1 tsp. at a time.

Indigestion: Take 2-3 "00" capsules of *Trikatu* (equal parts black pepper, Indian long pepper or as a substitute cayenne, and ginger powder) with a little warm water before meals. This is for lack of appetite, poor assimilation and malabsorption. For hyperacidity take 2-3 "00" capsules of equal parts gentian, barberry and licorice after meals.

Menstrual disorders: For cramps take 1 tbs. aloe vera gel with ¼ tsp. black pepper orally 3 times a day until cramps disappear. To promote menstruation take a tea of equal parts safflower and rose flowers, 1-2 tsps. per cup. For excessive menstruation take a tea of raspberry leaves and hibiscus flowers, 1-2 tsps. per cup.

Muscle Strain (upper body): An enema of 1 cup of calamus oil may be injected into the rectum. Retain for 30 minutes. For general muscle strain, apply warm ginger paste with turmeric (one tsp. of ginger with ½ tsp. of turmeric) to the affected area twice a day.

Nose Bleed: ½ tsp. chlorophyll plus 1 tsp. aloe vera gel mixed with 1 tsp. *ghee.* Take 3 times per day orally; or take 1 tbs. of bee pollen 2-3 times per day. Put ice on nose until bleeding stops.

Pain (external): Apply a ginger compress. To prepare a ginger compress, combine 2 tsps. of ginger powder with 1 tsp. of turmeric powder and add enough water to make a paste. Warm the paste and spread it evenly on a piece of gauze or cotton cloth. Then place the cloth on the affected area and apply a bandage over it. Keep it on overnight.

Poison bites and stings: Drink cilantro juice or apply sandalwood paste to the affected area; or drink an infusion of plantain, 1-2 tsps. per cup of water.

Poison (general): Take 1-2 tsps. *ghee* or 1 cup moderately strong licorice tea, and consult a medical practitioner.

Rash: Apply the pulp of cilantro leaf to the affected area or drink coriander tea (1 tsp. of coriander seeds to 1 cup of water).

Shock (fainting): Inhale fresh, broken onion, or inhale calamus root powder.

Sinus congestion: Inhale a pinch of calamus root powder or apply ginger paste to the affected area. One can also inhale the steam from a tea of ginger or eucalyptus leaves.

Sleep (lack of): Drink one cup of warm milk to which ½ tsp. nutmeg has been added. For more severe cases take an infusion of 1-2 tsp. valerian in a cup of water, to which 1 tsp. of *ashwagandha* powder can also be added if available. Massage the soles of the feet or the scalp with *brahmi* (gotu kola) oil, or alternatively, with warm sesame oil.

Sleep (excess): In the evening drink an infusion of ½ tsp. calamus root powder and ¼ tsp. ginger powder per cup of water; or, alternatively, drink a cup of basil leaf tea.

Sore Throat: Gargle with hot water mixed with ½ tsp. bayberry powder and ½ tsp. sage.

Sprain: Massage with equal parts of almond and garlic oil. In a hot water bath, add ½ cup of ginger powder and ½ cup of baking soda. To this add 1 tsp. of eucalyptus oil. Sit for 15 minutes.

Apply warm ginger paste with turmeric (1 tsp. of ginger with ½ tsp. of turmeric) to the affected area twice a day.

Swelling: Drink barley water: 4 parts of water boiled with 1 part of barley, then strain. Coriander tea also is beneficial. For external swelling, apply 2 parts of turmeric powder mixed with 1 part salt to the affected area. Drink gotu kola tea: 1 tbs. to 1 cup of water.

Toothache: Apply 3 drops of clove oil to the affected tooth.

APPENDIX IV

ENGLISH GLOSSARY

Alopecia	natural or abnormal baldness; loss of hair
Alterative	tending to restore normal health; cleanses and purifies the blood; alters existing nutritive and excretory processes gradually restoring normal body functions
Amenorrhea	absence or suppression of menstruation
Anabolic	constructive phase of metabolism; building up (repair and growth) of body substance
Analgesic	relieves pain
Anthelmintic	helps destroy and dispel parasites (includes vermides and vermifuges; in Ayurveda parasites include worms, bacteria, fungus and yeast)
Antibiotic	inhibits growth of or destroys microorganisms
Antipyretic	dispels heat, fire and fever
Antispasmodic	relieves spasms of voluntary and involuntary muscles
Aperient	a mild laxative
Aphrodisiac	reinvigorates the body by reinvigorating the sexual organs
Aromatic	herbs which contain volatile, essential oils which aid digestion and relieve gas
Astringent	firms tissues and organs; reduces discharges and secretions
Bitter tonic	bitter herbs which in small amounts stimulate digestion and otherwise help regulate fire in the body

Carminative	relieves intestinal gas, pain and distention; promotes peristalsis
Catabolic	destructive phase of metabolism
Cathartic	strong laxative which causes rapid evacuation
Demulcent	soothes, protects and nurtures internal membranes
Deobstruent	removes body obstructions
Diaphoretic	causes perspiration and increased elimination through the skin
Diuretic	promotes activity of kidney and bladder and increases urination
Dropsy	generalized edema
Dysmenorrhea	painful or difficult menstruation
Dyspnea	difficulty in breathing
Emetic	induces vomiting
Emmenagogue	helps promote and regulate menstruation
Emollient	soothes, softens and protects the skin
Enteritis	inflammation of the small intestine
Epistaxis	nosebleed
Erysipelas	an acute disease of skin and subcutaneous tissue with spreading inflammation and swelling
Expectorant	promotes discharge of phlegm and mucus from lungs and throat
Febrifuge	reduces fever
Gastritis	inflammation of the stomach
Hematemesis	vomiting of blood
Hemoptysis	spitting up of blood from the lungs or bronchial tubes
Hemostatic	stops the flow of blood; type of astringent that stops internal bleeding or hemorrhaging
Laxative	promotes bowel movements
Lithotriptic	substance that dissolves and discharges gall bladder and urinary stones and gravel
Malabsorption	inadequate absorption of nutrients from the intestinal tract

Menorrhagia	excessive bleeding during menstruation
Nephritis	inflammation of the kidney
Nervine	strengthens functional activity of nervous system; may be stimulants and sedatives
Neurasthenia	severe nerve weakness, nervous exhaustion
Nutritive tonic	increases weight and density and nourishes the body
Paroxymal fever	periodic, recurring fevers
Refrigerant	reduces body temperature and relieves thirst
Rejuvenative	prevents decay, postpones aging, revitalizes the organs
Sedative	calms or tranquilizes by lowering functional activity of organ or body part
Stimulant	increases internal heat, dispels internal chill and strengthens metabolism and circulation
Stomachic	strengthens stomach function
Suppuration	pus formation and discharge
Urticaria	skin condition characterized by itching welts; hives
Vasodilator	causes relaxation of the blood vessels
Vermicidal	kills parasites in the intestines
Vulnerary	assists in healing of wounds by protecting against infection and stimulating cell growth

APPENDIX V

SANSKRIT GLOSSARY

Agni	biological fire governing metabolism; cosmic force of transformation
Agni dipana	substances that increase *agni*, digestive fire
Ahamkara	ego; sense of separate self
Ama	toxins; undigested food or uneliminated waste materials
Ama pachana	substances that promote digestion or destruction of *Ama*
Anjana	herbal medicines applied to the eyes
Anupana	substances that serve as mediums for herbs to be taken with
Apana vayu	the *prana* governing downward movement of feces, urine, semen, menstrual fluid and birthing
Atman	The True Self or pure consciousness
Basti	medicated enema
Bhakti yoga	the yoga of devotion
Brahman	Spiritual reality, the Absolute
Buddhi	individualized cosmic intelligence; the power of determination
Chitta	conditioned consciousness in its totality
Dhatus	the seven basic tissue-elements of the body
Doshas	the three basic types of biological humors, which determine individual constitution

Guna	attribute; quality
Kapha	the bodily water humour
Mahat	cosmic intelligence
Manas	conditioned mind
Mantra	special seed-syllables that transmit cosmic energy
Nasya	administration of medicines through the nose
Nirama	without *ama*
Ojas	the subtle essence of all vital fluids, responsible for health, harmony and spiritual growth
Pancha karma	five types of purification or detoxification therapy
Pancha kashaya	five main methods of herbal preparation
Pitta	the bodily fire humour
Prabhava	special potencies of herbs apart from general rules
Prakruti	great nature; principle of creativity; matter
Prana	life-force; downward movement which governs inhalation and swallowing
Puja	devotional worship
Purusha	primal spirit; principle of sentience
Rajas	principle of energy, activity, emotion and turbulence
Rasa	initial taste of a substance; essence
Rasayana	rejuvenative therapy which regenerates body-mind, prevents decay, postpones aging
Sama	with *ama*
Samana	*Prana* that governs digestive system
Sattva	principle of light, perception, intelligence and harmony
Shakti	The Divine Energy/Cosmic Feminine principle
Shiva	The Divine Being/Cosmic Masculine principle
Soma	the essence energy of the mind and nervous system
Srotas	bodily channels

Tamas	principle of inertia, dullness, darkness and resistance
Tejas	fire of the mind
Udana	*Prana* that governs speech, energy, will, memory and exhalation
Vajikarana	substances that improve sexual vitality and functioning
Vata	the bodily air humour
Vedas	ancient scriptures of India
Vikruti	disease; deviation from nature
Vipaka	post-digestive effect (sweet, sour and pungent)
Virya	the energy of a substance as heating or cooling
Vyana	*Prana* that governs the circulatory sytem and movement of joints and muscles
Yantra	mystic diagrams; geometrical designs that manifest cosmic law and channel cosmic energy
Yoga	a methodology of the practical and coordinated application of knowledge; spiritually, the science of self-realization

APPENDIX VI

LATIN APPENDIX

Abutilon indicum	Atibala	Boerhaavia diffusa	Punarnava
Acacia senegal	Gum Arabic	Borago officinalis	Borage
Achillea millefolium	Yarrow	Boswellia thurifera	Frankincense
Acorus calamus	Calamus; Sweet Flag	Brassica alba	Mustard Seed
Adiandum capillus-veneris	Maidenhair Fern	Calendula officinalis	Calendula
Agrimonia eupatoria	Agrimony	Capsella bursapastoris	Shepherd's Purse
Allium cepa	Onion	Capsicum spp.	Cayenne and Paprika
Allium sativum	Garlic		
Aloe spp.	Aloe	Carbenia benedicta	Blessed Thistle
Alpinia officinarum	Galangal	Carthamus tinctorius	Safflower
Althea officinalis	Marshmallow	Carum carvi	Caraway
Amygdalus communis	Almond	Caryophyllus aromaticus	Cloves
Andrapogon muricatus	Vetiverian	Cassia acutifolia	Senna
Anethum graveolens	Dill	Caulophyllum thalictroides	Blue Cohosh
Angelica archangelica	Angelica	Ceanothus spp.	Red Root
Angelica sinensis	Tang Kuei	Cetraria islandica	Iceland Moss
Anthemis nobilis	Chamomile (Roman, Common)	Chenopodium anthelminticum	Wormseed
Apium graveolens	Wild Celery Seeds	Chimaphila umbellata	Pipsissewa
Apocynum androsaemifolium	Bitter Root	Chondrus crispus	Irish Moss
Aralia racemosa	Spikenard	Chrysanthemum indicum	Chrysanthemum
Arctium lappa	Burdock	Cichorium intybus	Chicory
Arctostaphylos uva-ursi	Uva Ursi; Bearberry	Cimicufuga racemosa	Black Cohosh
		Cinchona succirubra	Peruvian Bark
Arnica montana	Arnica	Cinnamomum camphora	Camphor
Artemesia absinthium	Wormwood	Citrus acida	Lime
Artemisia dracunculus	Tarragon	Citrus aurantium	Orange Peel
Artemesia vulgaris	Mugwort	Citrus limonum	Lemon
Asarum canadense	Wild Ginger	Cochlearia armoracia	Horseradish
Asclepias tuberosa	Pleurisy Root; Butterfly Weed	Collinsonia canadensis	Stoneroot
		Commiphora mukul	Guggulu
Asparagus officinalis	Asparagus	Coptis spp.	Gold Thread
Asparagus racemosus	Shatavari	Coriandrum sativum	Coriander (seed); Cilantro (fresh herb)
Avena sativa	Oat Straw		
Azadiracta indica	Neem; Nimba		
		Crataegus oxycantha	Hawthorn Berries
		Crocus Sativus	Saffron
Bambusa arundinaceae	Bamboo Manna; Vamsha Rochana	Cucurbita pepo	Pumpkin Seeds
		Cuminum cyminum	Cumin
Baptisia tinctoria	Indigo, Wild	Curcuma longa	Turmeric
Barosma betulina	Buchu	Cymbopogon citratus	Lemon Grass
Berberis spp.	Barberry	Cyperus rotundus	Nutgrass
Betula alba	Birch	Cypripedium pubescens	Lady's Slipper

Daucus carota	Wild Carrot	*Jasminum grandiflorum*	Jasmine
Dioscorea spp.	Wild Yam	*Jateorhize calumba*	Calumba
Dryopteris Felix-mas	Male Fern	*Juglans cinerea*	Butternut
		Juglans nigra	Walnut
Echinacea angustifolia	Echinacea	*Juniperus spp.*	Juniper Berries
Eclipta alba, etc.	*Bhringaraj*		
Elettaria cardamomum	Cardamom	*Larrea divaricata*	Chaparral
Eleuthrococus senticosus	Eleuthro;	*Laurus nobilis*	Bay Leaves
	Siberian Ginseng	*Lavandula spp.*	Lavender
Emblica officinalis	*Amla*	*Lawsonia spp.*	Henna
Ephedra vulgaris	Ma Huang; Ephedra	*Leonurus cardiaca*	Motherwort
Equisetum spp.	Horsetail	*Leptandra virginica*	Culver's Root;
Eriodictyon glutinosum	Yerba Santa		Black Root
Erythraea centaurium	Centaury, European	*Ligusticum porteri*	Osha
Eucalyptus globulus	Eucalyptus	*Lilum spp.*	Lily species
Euonymus atropurpureus	Wahoo	*Linum usitatissimum*	Flaxseed
Eupatorium perfoliatum	Boneset	*Lobelia inflata*	Lobelia
Eupatorium purpureum	Gravel Root	*Lythrum salicaria*	Purple
Euphrasia officinalis	Eyebright		Loosestrife
Euryale ferox	Chinese foxnuts;		
	Makhanna	*Mahonia repens*	Oregon Grape
		Malva spp.	Malva
Ferula asafoetida	Asafoetida; Hingu	*Marrubium vulgare*	Horehound
Foeniculum vulgaris	Fennel	*Matricaria chamomilla*	Chamomile
Fragaria spp.	Strawberry Leaves		(German)
Fucus visiculosis	Kelp	*Medicago sativa*	Alfalfa
		Melissa officinalis	Lemon Balm
Galium aparine	Cleavers	*Mentha arvensis*	Horsemint
Gaultheria procumbens	Wintergreen	*Mentha piperita*	Peppermint
Gentiana spp.	Gentian	*Mentha pulegium*	Pennyroyal
Geranium maculatum	Cranesbill;	*Mentha spicata*	Spearmint
	Wild Geranium	*Menyanthea trifoliata*	Buckbean;
Glycyrrhiza glabra	Licorice		Bogbean
Gossypium herbaceum	Cotton Root	*Mitchella repens*	Squaw vine
Grindelia spp.	Grindelia;	*Myristica fragrans*	Nutmeg; Mace
	Gumweed		
		Nardostachys jatamamsi	*Jatamamsi*
Hamamelis virginiana	Witch Hazel	*Nelumbo nucifera*	Lotus
Harpagophytum procumbens	Devil's Claw	*Nepeta cataria*	Catnip
Helonias dioica	False Unicorn		
Hibiscus rosa-sinensis	Hibiscus Flower	*Origanum marjorana*	Marjoram
Hordeum distichon	Barley	*Origanum vulgare*	Oregano
Humulus lupulus	Hops		
Hydrastis canadensis	Golden Seal	*Paeonia officinalis*	Peony
Hydrocotyl asiatica	Gotu Kola; *Brahmi*	*Panax ginseng*	Ginseng
Hypericum perforatum	St. John's Wort	*Papaver spp.*	Poppy
Hyssopus officinalis	Hyssop	*Passiflora incarnata*	Passion Flower
		Petroselinum spp.	Parsley
Ilex paraguayensis	Yerba Maté	*Phoenix dactylifera*	Date
Illicuim verum	Star Anise	*Picrorhiza Kurroa*	*Kutki*
Inula spp.	Elecampane	*Pimento officinalis*	Allspice
Ipomemea digitata	*Vidari Kanda*	*Pimpinella anisum*	Anise
Iris versicolor	Blue Flag	*Pinus alba*	White Pine
		Piper cubeba	Cubebs

Piper longum	*Pippali:* Indian Long Pepper	*Stellaria media*	Chickweed
Piper nigrum	Black Pepper	*Stillingia sylvatica*	Stillingia
Plantago major	Plantain	*Symphytum officinale*	Comfrey
Plantago psyllium	Psyllium Seed	*Symplocarpus foetidus*	Skunk Cabbage
Podophyllum peltatum	Mandrake, Amer.; Mayapple	*Tabebuia avellanedae*	Pau D'arco
Polygonatum spp.	Solomon's Seal	*Tamarindus indica*	Tamarind
Polygonum bistorta	Bistort	*Tanacetum vulgare*	Tansy
Polygonum multiflorum	Fo-ti	*Taraxacum officinale*	Dandelion
Populus tremuloides	White Poplar; Aspen	*Terminalia belerica*	*Bibhitaki*
		Terminalia chebula	*Haritaki*
Potentilla tormentilla	Tormentil	*Thymus vulgaris*	Thyme
Primula vulgaris	Primrose	*Tribulis terrestris*	*Gokshura*; Goathead; Puncture Vine
Prunella vulgaris	Self-Heal		
Prunus armeniaca	Apricot Seed	*Trifolium pratense*	Red Clover
Prunus spp.	Wild Cherry Bark	*Tussilago farfara*	Coltsfoot
Pueraria tuberosa	Kudzu	*Typha spp.*	Cattail
Punica granatum	Pomegranate		
		Ulmus fulva	Slippery Elm
Quercus alba	White Oak	*Urtica urens*	Nettle
Rehmannia glutinosa	Rehmannia	*Valeriana spp.*	Valerian
Rhamnus purshianus	Cascara Sagrada	*Verbascum thapsus*	Mullein
Rheum spp.	Rhubarb	*Verbena spp.*	Vervain
Rhus glabra, etc.	Sumach	*Viburnum opulus*	Crampbark
Ricinus communis	Castor Oil	*Viola spp.*	Violet
Rorippa nastrutium	Watercress	*Viscum album*	Mistletoe
Rosa spp.	Rose	*Vitis vinefera*	Grape
Rosmarinus officinalis	Rosemary		
Rubia cordifolia	*Manjishta*; Indian Madder	*Withania somnifera*	*Ashwagandha*; Winter Cherry
Rubus fructicosus, etc.	Blackberry	*Xanthoxylum spp.*	Prickly Ash
Rubus spp.	Raspberry	*Zea Mays*	Corn Silk
Rumex crispus	Yellow Dock	*Zingiber officinale*	Ginger
Ruta graveolens	Rue		
Sabbatia angularis	Centaury, American		
Saccharum granorum	Sugar (raw)		
Salix spp.	Willow Bark		
Salvia officinalis	Sage		
Salvia polystachya	Chia Seeds		
Sambucus spp.	Elder Flower		
Santalum albus	Sandalwood		
Sassafras officinale	Sassafras		
Satureia hortensis	Savory		
Scutellaria spp.	Skullcap		
Serenoa serrulata	Saw Palmetto		
Sesamum indicum	Sesame Seeds		
Sida cordifolia	*Bala*; India Country mallow		
Sida rhombifolia	*Mahabala*		
Smilax spp.	Sarsaparilla		
Stachys betonica	Betony, Wood		

SPECIAL AYURVEDIC AND CHINESE HERBS

ARJUNA   *Terminalia arjuna; Combretaceae*

(S) *Arjuna*

Part Used: bark
Energetics: astringent/cooling/pungent
PK– V+
Tissues: plasma, blood, muscle, bone, nerve
Systems: circulatory, digestive, nervous
Actions: heart tonic, circulatory stimulant, astringent, alterative, hemostatic
Indications: heart diseases of all types, angina, traumatic injury, broken bones, diarrhea, malabsorption, venereal diseases
Precautions: none noted
Preparation: powder (250 to 500 mg), decoction, herbal wine

ARJUNA is a close relative of the three herbs of the Triphala formula (*Haritaki, Amalaki and Bibhitaki*) and has a similar importance in Ayurvedic medicine as a tonic and rejuvenative agent. Its action is specific for the heart, and is useful in all types of heart diseases, promoting right heart function and aiding in longevity. *Arjuna* helps recovery after heart attacks, as well as helps in their prevention. It promotes healing of the soft tissue and of internal organs, and is specific for treating broken bones. It is a good blood thinner, while maintaining normal coagulation.

Today when heart disease is probably the main cause of death *Arjuna* is an important herb and can be taken as a general heart tonic for those with a propensity to heart attacks. On a psychological level *Arjuna* gives courage and strengthens the will, fortifying our heart to accomplish our true goals in life. It is often combined with other herbs for the heart like *Guggul*, *Gotu Kola* and *Ashwagandha*.

BAKUCHI   *Psoralea corylifolia; Leguminoseae*

(S) *Bakuchi*

(C) Bu Gu Zhi

Part Used: seed
Energetics: pungent, bitter/heating/pungent
      KV– P+
Tissues: plasma, blood
Systems: circulatory, urinary
Actions: alterative, diuretic, diaphoretic, rejuvenative, aphrodisiac, antiparasitical
Indications: impetigo, leucoderma, psoriasis, debility, round worms, chronic fevers, impotence, premature greying or falling out of the hair
Precautions: with *Pitta* should be balanced out with other more cooling herbs, avoid during chronic fevers
Preparation: powder (250 to 500 mg), oil

BAKUCHI is an excellent tonic and rejuvenative for the skin. It improves the complexion, restoring the luster to the skin and improving growth of nails and hair. It is good for rough, cracked, scaly skin and broken or brittle nails, such as are common in *Vata* constitutions and in the elderly. It helps eliminate discoloration of the skin, whether light or dark in color, and reestablishes normal skin tone. *Bakuchi* is considered to be the best herb for leucoderma and similar skin discolorations

Bakuchi oil applied topically for leucoderma helps stop the spread of discoloration and restores normal skin color. The oil is also good for folliculitis. *Psoralea* is also used for similar purposes in Chinese medicine where it is classified as a yang tonic or herb to improve primary vitality.

BILVA, Bael   Aegle marmelos; Rutaceae

(S) Bilva

Part Used: fruit (immature)
Energetics: astringent, sweet/cooling/sweet
        K– V+, increases Agni
Tissues: plasma, blood, fat, nerve
Systems: digestive, excretory, nervous
Actions: astringent, stomachic, digestive stimulant
Indications: malabsorption, chronic diarrhea (particularly in children), dysentery (amoebic), colic, diabetes, bleeding, cough, insomnia
Precautions: not used during acute fevers, safe in chronic fevers
Preparation: powder (250 mg to 1 gm), decoction, confection

BILVA is an important Ayurvedic astringent and stimulant for chronic weak digestion and malabsorption, improving both the digestive fire and small intestine function. Bilva is also one of the most sacred plants to Shiva, the God of Pure Consciousness, fortifying the heart and soothing the eyes. For those suffering from chronic loose stool and weak appetite its healing effects can be extraordinary.

One-half teaspoon of the powder along with one teaspoon of honey stops nausea and vomiting. One teaspoon of the powder mixed with enough goat's milk to make a paste is excellent for countering stomatitis and other ulcerative sores. Please note that the ripe fruit has laxative and nutritive properties and is not as astringent as the unripe fruit. Various jams and confections are made with the fruit.

BRAHMI   Hydrocotyle asiatica; Umbellifera
MANDUKA PARNI   Bacopa monniera; Scrophulariaceae

(S) Brahmi (what gives knowledge of Brahman or Supreme Reality), Manduka parni (what has the leaf of a frog)

Part used: root, plant
Energetics: bitter, astringent, sweet/cooling/sweet
        VPK=

Tissues: nerve, blood
Systems: nervous, muscular, circulatory, reproductive
Actions: brain tonic, sedative, antispasmodic, alterative, diuretic, astringent
Indications: anxiety, anger, insomnia, nerve pain, nervous debility, muscle spasms, paralysis, anemia, venereal diseases, weak immune system
Precautions: in large dosages may cause headaches or loss of consciousness, particularly in *Vata* constitutions
Preparation: powder (250 mg to 1 gm), decoction, juice

BRAHMI is perhaps the most important nervine herb used in Ayurvedic medicine. It revitalizes the brain cells, removing toxins and blockages within the nervous system, while at the same time having a nurturing effect. It improves memory and aids in concentration. Himalayan *Brahmi* is an important food for Yogis and improves meditation. A small amount of the fresh leaves are eaten daily for rejuvenating the mind. *Brahmi* helps awaken the crown chakra and balance the right and left hemispheres of the brain. It calms the heart and helps guard against heart attacks.

Brahmi helps us give up bad habits and addictions of all types. It aids in recovery from alcholism or drug abuse, and also helps us kick the sugar habit. For this reason it is added to many Ayurvedic formulas as a nervine and antispasmodic agent. It is cleansing to the blood, improves the immune system, allays excess sexual desire, and is excellent for venereal diseases, including AIDS. It cleanses the kidneys, while calming and soothing the liver.

Brahmi is one of the best herbs for balancing and rejuvenating *Pitta*, while at the same time strongly reducing *Kapha*. It can reduce *Vata* if taken in the proper dose or with other anti-*Vata* herbs, like *Ashwagandha*. A cup of *Brahmi* tea taken with honey before meditation is a great aid in the practice. As a milk decoction the herb is a good brain tonic, particularly if combined with *Ashwagandha*. Taken with basil and a little black pepper *Brahmi* is good for all kinds of fevers. As a rejuvenative it is best prepared in *ghee*. *Brahmi ghee* is an important medicine for the mind and heart that should be kept in every home.

There are several botanical controversies about *Brahmi*. First is the identity of *Brahmi* and a similarly used plant called *Manduka Parni* (*Bacopa*), which however is unrelated botanically. Generally the *Brahmi* (*Hydrocotyle*) is the preferable agent. Ayurveda, like many traditional systems, has emphasized using equivalent herbs because the same exact species is not always available everywhere in the country. This, however, can add to the botanical confusion. Several related plants to *Bacopa* grow in the Eastern United States.

The other controversy is about the identity of *Brahmi* and *Gotu Kola*. The two herbs are closely related botanically and possess similar properties (though *Gotu Kola* is a stronger diurectic and a weaker nervine). By recent accounts *Gotu Kola* is *Centella Asiatica* and so some Ayurvedic doctors do not like to simply identify the two. Because *Gotu Kola* is more readily available than *Brahmi* from India, and is not much different in properties, it is often used in its place.

CHITRAK   *Plumbago zeylonica*

(S) *Chitraka*

Part Used: root
Energetics: pungent/hot/pungent
　　　　　　　KV– P+ increases *Agni*
Tissues: blood, fat
Systems: digestive
Actions: stimulant, diaphoretic, carminative, emmenagogue, cholagogue
Uses: lack of appetite, indigestion, abdominal distention, hemorrhoids, edema, parasites, skin diseases, paralysis, mental disorders, arthritis
Precautions: use low dosages, large dosages can be toxic; do not take during pregnancy, urinary tract infections or bleeding disorders
Preparation: powder (250 to 500 mg)

Perhaps the best Ayurvedic herb for improving the digestive fire and increasing the digestive power of liver, spleen and small intestine, *Chitrak* often works even when hot spices like cayenne fail. It is better than *Trikatu* or *Asafoetida* and can be added to them for better results. Those suffering from chronic weak digestion and low appetite can benefit by taking this herb before or with meals. *Chitrak* aids in promotion of energy through proper digestion and assimilation. It stimulates the liver to digest fats and sugars as well. Taken with *Shilajit*, *Chitrak* serves as an excellent weight regulator.

GARCINIA CAMBODIA

Part Used: root, fruit
Energetics: pungent, bitter/cooling/pungent
        PK– V+
Tissues: fat, nerve
Systems: digestive, nervous, muscular
Actions: sedative, antispasmodic
Indications: obesity, anxiety, insomnia, nerve pain, muscle spasms
Precautions: high *Vata* conditions
Preparation: powder (250 to 500 mg), extract

Much modern research has shown this herb and its active ingredients to be one of the best remedies for weight reduction. *Garcinia* aids in fat metabolism, lowers the appetite, and helps reduce the mental and emotional addiction to food and sugar. While an Ayurvedic herb it is not commonly used in traditional formulas.

GUDUCHI (Amrit) *Tinospora cordifolia; Menispermaceae*

(S) *Guduchi, Amrita (Ambrosia)*

(C) Kuan Jin Teng

Part Used: stem and root, powdered bitter starchy extract
Energetics: bitter, astringent, sweet/hot/sweet
        VPK=
Tissues: blood, fat, reproductive
Systems: circulatory, digestive, reproductive
Actions: bitter tonic, febrifuge, alterative, diuretic, aphrodisiac, rejuvenative, antirheumatic
Indications: fever, convalescence from febrile diseases, malaria, hyperacidity, hepatitis, jaundice, diabetes, heart disease, tuberculo-

sis, arthritis, gout, skin diseases, hemorrhoids
Precautions: use with care during pregnancy
Preparation: powder (250 to 500 mg), extract (*Guduchi or Giloy Sattva*)

Guduchi is a rejuvenative for *Pitta* and powerful nutritive herb to take during recovery periods from fevers or infectious diseases. Its hot nature is anti-*Ama*, not *Pitta* aggravating and destroys toxins without aggravating heat or fire in the body. *Guduchi*, like *Ashwagandha* and *Shatavari*, is an excellent tonic for the immune system, and therefore one of the best herbs for poor immune function. It is particularly important for countering chronic low grade fevers or difficult to treat infections from Epstein bar virus to AIDS, such as many people today suffer from. It increases our positive energy in conditions of debility like chronic fatigue syndrome.

The bitter starch which comes from the plant, called *Guduchi* or *Giloy Sattva* is the best way to take it. Taken with ghee *Guduchi* reduces *Vata*, with sugar it reduces *Pitta*, and with honey it reduces *Kapha*. The Chinese use the herb mainly for swelling owing to arthritis or traumatic injury.

GURMAR *Gymnena sylvestre; Asclepiadaceae*

(S) *Meshasringi, Shardunika, Madhunashini* (what destroys the sweet taste)

Part Used: leaves
Energetics: astringent, pungent/heating/pungent
KV– P=
Tissues: blood, plasma
Systems: digestive, circulatory
Actions: astringent, digestive stimulant, diuretic
Indications: diabetes, obesity, hypoglycemia, kidney stones, enlargement of liver and spleen
Precautions: none noted
Preparation: powder (250 mg to 1 gm)

GURMAR counters our craving for sugar, dulling the taste buds, and soothing the nerves. It helps control the appetite and reduce sugar cravings. It calms and soothes the liver and pancreas. A little of the powder taken in the mouth renders a person temporarily insensitive to sugar. A wonderful herb for those seeking to reduce their sugar dependency, *Gurmar* is particularly useful during the initial onset of diabetes and can prevent the disease from developing. A little taken when sugar cravings arise prevents them from developing further.

JATAMAMSI   *Nardostachys jatamansi; Valerianaceae*

(S) *Jatamamsi*

Part Used: root
Energetics: bitter, astringent, sweet/cooling/sweet
          VPK=
Tissues: nerve, blood
Systems: nervous, muscular, circulatory
Actions: brain tonic, sedative, antispasmodic, analgesic, anti-inflammatory, emmenagogue
Indications: anxiety, insomnia, headache, nerve pain, muscle spasms, colic, cramps, menopause, palpitations, hysteria
Precautions: none noted
Preparation: powder (250 to 1 gm), oil

JATAMAMSI has a special quality (*Prabhava*) to treat mental and psychological diseases, helping us deal with emotional turbulence and subconscious traumas. It is perhaps the best and safest Ayurvedic sedative, similar to its relative *Valerian* in properties but safer and more balancing in its effect, calming but not dulling the way *Valerian* sometimes is. Unlike *Valerian*, which is heating, *Jatamamsi* is cooling and helps soothe the overheated mind and inflamed nerves. Combined with *Ashwagandha* it makes an excellent brain tonic and memory improving agent. *Jatamamsi* can be added to herbal formulas wherever a sedative, analgesic or antispasmodic is required.

For poor memory boil one teaspoon of *Jatamamsi* in one cup of warm milk for five minutes and drink in the early morning (add some sugar or cardamom to help improve the taste if you wish). One-half teaspoon *Jatamamsi* in one teaspoon of honey applied externally serves to beautify the skin.

KAPIKACCHU   *Mucuna pruriens; Papilionaceae*

(S) *Kapikacchu, Atmagupta, Vanari*

Part Used: seed
Energetics: bitter, sweet/warm/sweet
       KV– P=
Tissues: reproductive, nerve
Systems: nervous, reproductive, respiratory
Actions: tonic, rejuvenative, aphrodisiac, astringent
Indications: general debility, sexual debility, impotence, infertility, leucorrhea, spermatorrhea, asthma, nervous debility, paralysis, Parkinson's disease
Precautions: menstrual bleeding, menorrhagia
Preparation: powder (250 mg to 1 gm), milk decoction, confections

The seeds of this plant are one of the best tonics and aphrodisiacs to the reproductive system, male or female. They increase sexual energy, strengthen the reproductive organs and through them vitalize our entire system. They are commonly used with *Amalaki, Ashwagandha, Shatavari, Bala, Vidari, Gokshura* and other tonics to make various pills and herbal jellies. While *Kapikacchu* is one of the more expensive Ayurvedic herbal tonics, it is still far less expensive than ginseng and many other herbal tonics. A not unpleasant tasting bean, *Kapikacchu* can be cooked in rice as a wonderful herbal food.

One teaspoon of the seeds boiled in one cup of water stimulates sexual energy and prevents premature ejaculation. For bronchial asthma, one-half teaspoon of the powder along with a teaspoon of ghee serves as a good bronchodialator. *Kapikacchu* has recently been found to be a natural source of L-dopa, used to treat Parkinson's disease. Several Ayurvedic companies in India use an extract of the herb for this purpose. It can be taken as a regular herbal food, one to two teaspoons a day, for Parkison's and similar diseases of nerve weakness.

KATUKA (Kutki)   Picrorrhiza kurroa
(S) *Katuka*

(C) Hu Huang Lian

Part Used: root
Energetics: bitter, pungent/cold/pungent
          KP– V=
Tissues: plasma, blood, fat
System: digestive, circulatory, urinary
Actions: bitter tonic, antipyretic, alterative, laxative, antibiotic
Uses: fever, cough, hepatitis, asthma, bronchitis, parasites, toxic
blood conditions, eye inflammations, obesity, diabetes
Precautions: high *Vata* (air) conditions, severe debility, hypoglyce-
mia
Preparation: powder (250 to 500 mg), decoction, tincture, ghee

KATUKA is probably the most commonly used Ayurvedic bitter
tonic and has a place like *Golden Seal* in the natural medicine of
India. It counters fevers, infections and any type of bacterial
inflammation, and aids in detoxification of the blood. It is a good
tonic to the liver, spleen, small intestine and other *Pitta* systems.
Along with other bitter tonics like *Gentien* or *Barberry*, *Katuka* is
excellent for improving digestion and stimulating the flow of
hydrochloric acid in the stomach.

One-half teaspoon of *Katuka*, along with one teaspoon honey and
one teaspoon aloe vera gel taken three times a day is an excellent
tonic for improving liver function. One-half teaspoon of *Katuka*
along with one-half teaspoon of *Vidanga* taken with one teaspoon
of honey twice a day before meals helps eliminate pinworms and
thread worms. One-half teaspoon of *Katuka* along with an equal
amount of *Turmeric* taken before meals regulates blood sugar in
diabetic patients.

KUTAJ (Kurchi) *Holarrhena antidysenterica; Apocynaceae*

(S) *Kutaja*

Part Used: bark, root and seed

Energetics: astringent, bitter/cold/pungent
 PK– V+
Tissues: blood, muscle
Systems: digestive, excretory, circulatory
Actions: astringent, anthelmintic, amoebicidal
Indications: diarrhea and dysentery (both acute and chronic),
colitis, parasites, malabsorption, hemorrhoids, menorrhagia
Precautions: constipation
Preparation: powder (250 to 500 mg), decoction, herbal wine

KUTAJ is the main Ayurvedic herb for bacterial or amoebic
dysentery; hence a good herb to know of if one travels in India or
other third world countries, where travelers easily come down with
such conditions. *Kutaj* is specific to the colon in its action and
helps restore normal colon function. It is excellent for conditions
like candida that are based upon poor flora in the intestines.
However, owing to its strong nature, it should not be taken over
long periods of time. Today *Kutaj* usually comes in a brown form
but a white form also exists but is harder to get.

For bleeding hemorrhoids take one-half teaspoon of *Kutaj* in one-
half cup of pomegranate juice, two or three times a day to stop the
bleeding. For burning urination take one-half teaspoon of *Kutaj*
boiled for five minutes in one cup of milk two or three times a day.

LODHRA   *Symplocos racemosa; Styraceae*

(S) *Lodhra*

Part Used: bark
Energetics: bitter, astringent/cold/pungent
 PK– V+
Tissues: blood
Systems: circulatory, menstrual
Actions: astringent, hemostatic, alterative, diuretic
Indications: excess menstrual bleeding, uterine hemorrhage,
inflammatory diseases of the eye, diarrhea, dysentery, edema
Precautions: amenorrhea
Preparation: powder (250 to 500 mg), decoction

LODHRA is an important astringent and menstrual regulator and a significant Ayurvedic hemostatic, much like *Manjistha (Madder)*. It helps prevent miscarriages and strengthens the fetus. *Lodhra* is found in many Ayurvedic women's formulas. A tea made of equal parts *Lodhra* and *Sandalwood* is good for excessive menstrual bleeding. The herb is found in many Ayurvedic tooth powders as well. A mouthwash made of a teaspoon of *Lodhra* powder with a pinch of *Alum* is good for receding gums and sensitive teeth.

PHYLLANTHUS   *Phyllanthus Niruri; Euphorbiaceae*

(S) *Bhumyamalaki*

Part Used: plant
Energetics: bitter, astringent, sweet/cooling/pungent
          VPK=
Tissues: bone, plasma, blood
Systems: circulatory, digestive, skeletal
Actions: alterative, cholagogue, vulnerary, anti-inflammatory, diuretic
Indications: hepatitis, jaundice, liver and spleen diseases, skin rashes, itch, venereal diseases, diabetes, anemia
Precaution: high *Vata*
Preparation: powder (250 mg to 1 gm), poultice (externally)

PHYLLANTHUS is one of the best Ayurvedic herbs for the liver, and one of the few that has had success in treating both chronic and acute hepatitis. In this era of liver toxicity it is an excellent liver tonic and rejuvenative. It helps deal with the side effects of alcohol, tobacco, drugs and liver damaging chemicals. Such an herb naturally has a potential widespread application.

PUNARNAVA   *Boerhaavia diffusa; Nyctaginaceae*

(S) *Punarnava* (what renews us)

Part Used: plant
Energetics: bitter, sweet/heating/pungent
          KV– P+
Tissues: plasma, blood

Systems: urinary, circulatory
Actions: alterative, blood tonic, diuretic, rejuvenative
Indications: anemia, edema, difficult or burning urination, kidney stones, heart disease, alcoholism, hepatitis, hemorrhoids
Precautions: dehydration
Preparation: powder (250 to 500 mg), decoction

PUNARNAVA literally means the plant that makes one new again and has a special power to renew our health and vitality. It rebuilds the blood and strengthens the kidneys, improving their function and through revitalizing this key organ, aids in our overall health and vitality. *Punarnava* is particularly good for conditions of weak kidney function leading to water retention and edema. As a tonifying diuretic it is often combined with *Gokshura*.

SALLAKI   *Boswellia seffata; Burseraceae*

(S) *Sallaki*

Part Used: resin
Energetics: bitter, sweet, astringent/cooling/pungent
             VPK=
Tissues: blood, muscle, fat, reproductive
Systems: circulatory, muscular, skeletal
Actions: alterative, antispasmodic, analgesic
Indications: arthritis, rheumatism, gout, nerve pain, muscle spasms
Precaution: none noted
Preparation: purified powder (250 mg to 1 gm)

SALLAKI is a resin related to *Guggul* and *Myrrh* and used for similar purposes of cleansing the blood and countering arthritic pain. It also aids in the healing of soft tissue injuries. Its cooling nature makes it particularly good for inflamed and swollen joints where there is some *Pitta* involvement.

SHANKHA PUSHPI   *Evoluvus alsinodes*

(S) *Shankha pushpi*

Part Used: plant, juice

Energetics: astringent/warm/sweet
        VPK=
Tissues: nerve
Systems: nervous, circulatory
Actions: nervine, sedative, brain tonic
Indications: nervous debility, mental or emotional exhaustion, epilepsy, insomnia, insanity
Precautions: none noted
Preparation: powder (250 mg to 1 gm), decoction

Shankha pushpi is one of the most important Ayurvedic nervines along with *Brahmi, Calamus* and *Jatamamsi.* In fact it is often considered to be the best of these. *Shankha pushpi* is excellent for nerve pain, particularly that owing to cold or debility. It improves memory, concentration and perception, and aids in the rejuvenation of the mind. It increases circulation to the brain and stimulates our higher cerebral functions, improving our overall intelligence and creativity. *Sarasvata churna,* a powder prepared with herb, is widely used in attention deficit disorder and helps prevent loss of memory.

SHILAJIT

(S) *Shilajita*

Energetics: astringent, pungent, bitter/warm/pungent
        KV– P+
Tissues: nerve, reproductive
Systems: urinary, nervous, reproductive
Actions: alterative, diuretic, lithotriptic, antiseptic, tonic, rejuvenative
Indications: diabetes, obesity, jaundice, gall stones, dysuria, cystitis, edema, kidney stones, hemorrhoids, sexual debility, menstrual disorders, asthma, epilepsy, insanity, skin diseases, parasites
Precautions: not for febrile diseases
Preparation: pill, powder (250 to 500 mg)

SHILAJIT is one of the wonder medicines of Ayurveda, used for many conditions of weakness and debility. It is not an herb but a kind of natural mineral pitch from the Himalayas and carries the healing power of these great mountains. There are several varieties of the substance, of which the black color has the main therapeutic properties. It can be expensive but does not require large dosages.

Shilajit possesses great curative powers and is considered capable of treating many diseases, particularly those of the aging process. It is an important rejuvenative and tonic particularly for *Kapha*, *Vata*, and the kidneys, as in the case of people who have long suffered from diabetes and asthma. It can be taken for general health maintenance and is good for those who do much mental work or practice yoga. The Ayurvedic jelly *Chyavanprash* contains *Shilajit* as one of its main ingredients. It acts as a catalytic agent for promoting the action of other tonic agents.

VIDANGA   *Embelia ribes; Myrsinaceae*

Part Used: fruit
Energetics: pungent, astringent/warm/pungent
          KV– P+
Tissue: blood, fat
Systems: digestive, excretory
Actions: anthelmintic, carminative, laxative, expectorant
Indications: worms (tape, round, ring), obesity
Precautions: sexual debility
Preparation: powder (250 mg to 1 gm), decoction

VIDANGA is the most important Ayurvedic herb for eliminating parasites and treating worms of all types. It improves the function of the large intestine and helps restore its ability to eliminate toxins. It is also useful for weight reduction and helps control the appetite.

WHITE MUSALI   *Safet musli*
                              Asparagus adscendens; Liliaceae

Part Used: root
Energetics: sweet/cool/sweet
          PV– K+ (in excess)

Tissues: reproductive, fat, all tissues in general
Systems: reproductive, respiratory
Actions: nutritive tonic, demulcent, diurectic, galactagogue
Indications: general and sexual debility, infertility, impotence,
diarrhea, leticorrhea, spermatorrhea
Precautions: Ama and congestive disorders
Preparation: powder (250 mg to 1 gm), milk decoction, confec-
tions

WHITE MUSALI is a relative of Shatavari, with which it is often
combined. The herb is an excellent building and revitalizing tonic
for wasting diseases and tissue deficiency in general. Specifically it
strengthens the reproductive system and increases reproductive
tissue, for either male or female. It is good during pregnancy for
nourishing the fetus and postpartum for promoting the production
and flow of breast milk. One-half teaspoon of the herb along with
one-half teaspoon of Shatavari can be boiled for five minutes in a
cup of milk and taken morning and evening for this purpose.

BOTANICAL INDEX

GENERAL INDEX

BIBLIOGRAPHY

A BAREFOOT DOCTOR'S MANUAL. Seattle, WA: Cloudburst Press, 1977.

Bensky Dan, Andrew Gamble. comp. & eds. *CHINESE HERBAL MEDICINE, MATERIA MEDICA*. Seattle, WA: Eastland Press, 1986.

Bhishagratna, K. L. trans. *SUSHRUTA SAMHITA*. Varanasi, India: Chowkhamba Sanskrit Series, 1981.

Christopher, John R. *SCHOOL OF NATURAL HEALING*. Provo, Utah, BiWorld, 1976.

Dash, Bhagwan, Mandred Junius. *A HAND BOOK OF AYURVEDA*. New Delhi, India: Concept Publishing Company, 1983.

Dash, Bhagwan, Lalitesh Kashyap. *MATERIA MEDICA OF AYURVEDA*. New Delhi, India: Concept Publishing Co., 1980.

Hutchens, Alma R. *INDIAN HERBOLOGY OF NORTH AMERICA*. Windsor, Ontario: Merco, 1974.

Lad, Vasant. *AYURVEDA: THE SCIENCE OF SELF-HEALING*. Twin Lakes, WI: Lotus Press, 1984.

Moore, Michael. *MEDICINAL PLANTS OF THE MOUNTAIN WEST*. Santa Fe, NM: The Museum of New Mexico Press, 1982.

Nadkarni, K. M. *INDIAN MATERIA MEDICA*. Bombay, India: Popular Prakasham, 1976.

Savnur, H. V. *AYURVEDIC MATERIA MEDICA*. Delhi, India: Sri Satguru Publications, 1984.

Sharma, D. P. *TREATISE ON THIRTY IMPORTANT BAIDYANATH AYURVEDIC PRODUCTS*. Patna, India: Shree Baidyanath Ayurved Bhawan Ltd., 1977.

Sharma, R. K., Bhagwan Dash, trans., *CHARAK SAMHITA*. Varanasi, India: Chowkhamba Sanskrit Series, 1977.

Tierra, Michael. *THE WAY OF HERBS*. New York, NY: Washington Square Press, 1983.

ABOUT THE AUTHORS

DR. VASANT LAD M.A.Sc., brings a wealth of classroom and practical experience to the United States. A native of India, he served for three years as Medical Director of the Ayurveda Hospital in Pune, India. He also held the position of Professor of Clinical Medicine at the Pune University College of Ayurvedic Medicine where he instructed for 15 years. Dr. Lad's academic and practical training included the study of allopathy (Western Medicine) and surgery as well as traditional Ayurveda. Beginning in 1979, he has traveled throughout the United States sharing his knowledge of Ayurveda, and in 1984, he returned to Albuquerque as Director of the Ayurvedic Institute.

Dr. Lad is also the author of AYURVEDA, THE SCIENCE OF SELF HEALING and many published articles on various aspects of Ayurveda. He presently directs the Ayurvedic Institute in Albuquerque and teaches the three semester Ayurvedic Studies Certificate Program. Dr. Lad also travels extensively in North America throughout the year, consulting privately and giving seminars on Ayurveda; history, theory, principles and practical applications.

THE AYURVEDIC INSTITUTE, ALBUQUERQUE, NM

Founded in 1984, the Ayurvedic Institute was established to promote an understanding of Ayurveda, probably the oldest system of total health (mental, physical and spiritual) known to man.
THE INSTITUTE offers certificate courses, seminars including Jyotisha and Sanskrit, a correspondence course in Ayurveda and membership which includes the quarterly journal "Ayurveda Today".
THE WELLNESS CENTER, incorporated within the Institute, offers consultations with Dr. Lad in person and over the phone, Pancha Karma and other Ayurvedic Treatments.
THE HERB DEPARTMENT, dispenses herbs and herbal compounds as well as Ayurvedic tinctures, oils and other products. Books pamphlets, audio and video tapes on Ayurveda are also available.

THE AYURVEDIC INSTITUTE
11311 Menaul NE
Albuquerque, NM 87112
(505) 291-9698

ABOUT THE AUTHORS

DR. DAVID FRAWLEY (PANDIT VAMADEVA SHASTRI) is one of the few Westerners recognized in India as a Vedic teacher (Vedacharya). His many fields of expertise include Ayurvedic medicine, Vedic Astrology, Yoga, Vedanta and the Vedas themselves. He is the author of over twenty books on these subjects, including half a dozen books on Ayurveda. His Ayurvedic books address the issues of Ayurvedic herbalism, Ayurvedic psychology, Ayurveda and Yoga, and the Ayurvedic treatment of common diseases, offering a full range of information on both Ayurvedic theory and practice. He has also written many articles for different newspapers, magazines and journals, and has taught and lectured throughout the world, including India.

Dr. Frawley was regarded as one of the twenty-five most influential Yoga teachers in America today according to the *Yoga Journal*. *The Indian Express*, one of India's largest English language newspapers, recently called him "a formidable scholar of Vedanta and easily the best known Western teacher of the Vedic wisdom." *India Today*, the *Time Magazine* of India, has called him, "Certainly America's most singular practicing Hindu."

Currently Dr. Frawley is the director of the American Institute of Vedic Studies and the president of the American Council of Vedic Astrology (ACVA). He is on the editorial board for the magazine *Yoga International*. The American Institute of Vedic Studies features his correspondence courses on Ayurveda and on Vedic Astrology.

American Institute of Vedic Studies

The American Institute of Vedic Studies is an educational and research center devoted to Vedic and Yogic knowledge. It teaches related aspects of Vedic Science including Ayurveda, Vedic Astrology, Yoga, Tantra and Vedanta with special reference to their background in the Vedas. It offers books, articles, correspondence courses and longer training programs. The Institute is engaged in educational projects in the greater field of Hindu Dharma.

Long term projects include:
- Ayurvedic Psychology and Yoga: The mental and spiritual aspect of Ayurveda relative to Raja Yoga and Vedanta.
- Medical Astrology: Relative to both health and disease for body and mind.
- Translations and interpretations of the Vedas, particularly the Rig Veda, and an explication of the original Vedic Yoga.
- Vedic History: The history of India and of the world from a Vedic perspective and also as reflecting latest archaeological work in India.
- Vedic Europe: Explaining the connections between the Vedic and ancient European cultures and religions.
- Mantra Yoga and the meaning of the Sanskrit alphabet.
- Redefining Vedic and Hindu knowledge in a modern context for the coming millennium.

The Institute has helped found various organizations including the California College of Ayurveda, the American Council of Vedic Astrology, the World Association for Vedic Studies, and the British Association of Vedic Astrology. It is in contact with related organizations worldwide. For further information contact:

American Institute of Vedic Studies
PO Box 8357, Santa Fe, NM 87504-8357
Ph: 505-983-9385; Fax: 505-982-5807
Dr. David Frawley (Pandit Vamadeva Shastri), Director
Web: www.vedanet.com   Email: vedanet@aol.com